Vegan I...

Vegan Diet and Intermittent Fasting for Rapid Weight Loss, Reset & Cleanse Your Body, Nutrion Guide for Beginners with ketogenic approach, Meal Plan with Cookbook & Recipes.

[Dr. John Tortora]

COPYRIGHT

CONTENTS

Recipe Index

Introduction

The ketogenic diet is now more popular than ever. This lifestyle, which was originally developed in order to treat chronic and neurological illnesses, has been found to boost weight loss while increasing energy. However, many vegans and those on the plant-based lifestyle who may want to benefit from these aspects of the ketogenic diet may be wary if they can consume a diet that is both vegan and low in carbohydrates. In this book, you will learn exactly how to maintain healthy vegan ketosis, which will allow you to gain health, lose weight, increase energy, decrease hunger, and decrease your carbon footprint. A healthy, satisfying, and tasty ketogenic diet doesn't have to include bacon and cheese when instead you can enjoy delicious treats made with avocados, nuts, seeds, tofu, and more!

The ketogenic diet has been proven to not only treat neurological conditions, such as epilepsy, but it can also treat diabetes, insulin resistance, excessive weight gain, poly-cystic ovary syndrome, Alzheimer's disease, multiple sclerosis, and even cancer in some cases! These benefits are boosted by the addition of the vegan diet, which has long been shown to decrease aging and increase longevity. There is no reason to settle for poor health, rapid aging, and lagging energy when you can easily maintain a delicious and healthy lifestyle which will increase your overall quality of life while allowing you to still eat many of your favorite dishes.

By the time you finish this book, you will have full confidence in your ability to easily maintain a balanced vegan ketogenic diet complete with menu planning, prepping, and a number of recipes to get you well on your way to success.

Chapter 1:

Veganism 101

The vegan lifestyle is more than a simple diet. By taking up veganism you are making a choice for upholding ethical and moral standards in the animal-farming industries, lessening your carbon footprint on the planet, and making strides for improved health. All of these benefits have been proven by science, as there have been countless studies on the effects of the vegan lifestyle. This is especially important, as the consumption of meat in the Western world is only increasing. Since the year 2017, the demand for meat-based products has increased by a shocking nine-hundred and eighty-seven percent! With the consumption of meat on the rise, so too is climate change, animal abuse by corporations, and preventable diseases.

Thankfully, more people are taking steps to become vegans more than ever. Between 2012 and 2017 the number of people interested and Googling veganism quadrupled. The number of resources available to make the vegan lifestyle simple has made this a choice much easier to make. You no longer have to worry about whether the vegan diet is "possible," as it has been proven to be true. It is now possible to find vegan ingredients and meal options at the grocery store, restaurants, catered events, and even fast-food joints.

However, veganism is more than avoiding meat. It is a lifestyle in which people choose to avoid all products made with meat, dairy, eggs, or other animal by-products such as gelatin and collagen. The one subject that is up to debate between many vegans is whether honey and beeswax should be avoided. While purists choose to avoid any bee products, some vegans believe that these do not cause harm or cruelty to bees, and therefore include them on their diet. Therefore, it is up to your individual preferences whether or not you use beeswax products such as certain natural chap-sticks, lipsticks, and soaps. Although, honey should generally be avoided on the vegan ketogenic diet, as honey is high in natural sugars and carbohydrates.

The Health Benefits of Veganism

There are many health benefits of the vegan lifestyle. In fact, there are so many that we are unable to cover all of the benefits within this book. However, let's explore some of the more common benefits, especially those that treat symptoms and illnesses that are especially detrimental and prevalent in modern society. For instance, a study published in 2007 revealed that when Westerners consume a vegetarian diet they have lower rates of cholesterol, gallstones, constipation, and appendicitis. They also experience decreased body fat and a lower risk of death caused by ischemic heart disease. These statistics were all compared to Westerners who did consume meat products, proving that a plant-based lifestyle really does make the difference.

Now that you have a general idea of some of the health benefits the vegan lifestyle includes, let's have a look into some of the specifics.

Weight Loss:
While the reduced risk of diseases, and the possibility to even manage a disease you already have, is always a good reason to try a new lifestyle, many people are also looking for weight loss. There is nothing wrong with being fat, but that does not change the fact that it can increase your risk of disease. Many people hope to lose weight in order to become more active, reduce their risk of disease, feel better in their daily lives, and feel more comfortable in their own skin. Whatever your reason for losing weight, you will be happy to know that the vegan ketogenic diet can help. In a study by the European Association for the Study of Diabetes the diet of vegetarians and vegans was compared to that of carnivorous non-vegetarians. While this study was largely initiated to study the link between diet and diabetes, it was also found that by choosing a vegan lifestyle people can increase their metabolism, reduce fat located around the muscles, and help people to lose weight in a more effective manner. This will help people to lose overall body fat while also decreasing their risk of developing type II diabetes.

In another study, people on the National Education Program's diet and the vegan diet were compared for a period of two years. Throughout the course of the study, it was found that the people on a vegan diet, compared to the NCEP diet, lost a more significant amount of weight.

Diabetes:
The larger a study is the more reliable and accurate the results. This is good news when it comes to a Canadian-American study on the effects of veganism and diabetes, as this study used the combined efforts of over forty-one thousand participants. Specifically, twenty-six thousand women participated in and fifteen-thousand men. These participants came from various lifestyles, demographics, and diets. When sorting the participants the scientists placed them in groups of people who were on omnivorous, pescetarian, semi-vegetarian, Lacto-Ovo vegetarian, and vegan diets. This study was in place for two years, after which the participants filled out a questionnaire to determine their health after being on their given diets for a time. The results found that the vegan group had the lowest

risk of developing diabetes, with only 0.54% developing the disease after the two years. On the other hand, those on the omnivorous diet developed diabetes at a significantly increased risk, at 2.12%. Overall, with all of the food groups taken into account, it was found that the fewer animal-based products a person consumed the lower their risk of developing diabetes.

Heart Disease:
The vegan ketogenic diet is able to greatly benefit heart disease. This is due to the promotion of heart-healthy fats and low-carbohydrate/high-fiber foods. These foods have been proven to decrease the risk of heart disease, promoting overall heart health and longevity.
A study conducted at Oxford University analyzed the effects of various diets on elven-thousand participants. These included omnivorous, pescetarian, vegetarian, and vegan diets. Each of these diets resulted in drastically different rates of blood pressure, with those on the omnivorous diet having the highest average blood pressure and those on the vegan diet having the lowest average blood pressure.
Similarly, another study found that meat eaters have the highest cholesterol whereas vegans have the lowest cholesterol, with pescatarian and vegetarians being between the two groups. The same study found that people who have chosen life-long vegan lifestyles have a fifty-seven percent reduced risk of developing heart disease, whereas vegetarians only have a twenty-four percent reduced risk. Yes, a decrease in twenty-four percent is significant, but when vegans have a decreased risk of over twice that you have to acknowledge that the only contributing factor isn't meat. Along with avoiding meat, it is also vital to avoid dairy and eggs.

Cancer:
One of the leading causes of death in the world is cancer. There are many types, which can hide within the body until it becomes nearly impossible to treat. If you don't catch cancer early, then it is all too easy for it to overtake the body. Thankfully, there are ways you can decrease your risk of developing this devastating disease. In fact, one of the most reliable

organizations, the World Health Organization (W.H.O), has found that one-third of cancer cases can be prevented with our choices. This doesn't mean people are to blame for developing cancer, however, it does mean that if you make choices now you will have a decreased risk of developing it in the future. For instance, studies have found that be consuming the recommended seven portions of fruits and vegetables a day you can decrease your mortality risk from cancer by fifteen percent.

Soy products are frequently consumed on the vegan diet, which is also a great choice on the keto vegan diet due to their low-carb contents. A study on breast cancer analyzed the diets of over a thousand Asian-American women, especially those from the Japanese, Chinese, and Filipino cultures. This study found that the more a person consumes soy products the more significantly they are at a reduced risk of developing breast cancer. Specifically, those who consumed soy products at least once a week both during adolescence and adulthood were at the lowest risk of developing this devastating cancer.

How does the vegan diet have so many health benefits? Sure, avoiding animal-based products is a large part of the equation, but it goes beyond this. In fact, many people believe that the increase in phytochemicals found in plant-based foods is a large contributing factor in the benefits. By combining these two elements together the vegan lifestyle is a powerful diet that can overcome many of today's deadliest illnesses.

Studies have found that our consumption of plant-based foods greatly decreases our risk of developing many diseases, including the top causes of death in the modern world. For instance, heart disease, Alzheimer's disease, stroke, cancer, diabetes, and neurodegenerative diseases can all be prevented or reduced with the increase of healthy plant foods and the phytonutrients they contain.

However, while many of us know about vitamins and minerals within foods, what are phytochemicals? There are over the five-thousand bioactive matter that greatly impacts our overall health and risk of developing or contracting the disease. Sadly, with current technology, there is still much left unknown about phytochemicals. In fact, scientists believe there may be additional three-thousand types of phytochemicals that have yet to be identified. Thankfully, with the increase in scientific understanding and advancement more is beginning to be understood of phytochemicals and their role in human health. For instance, scientists now know that they are a large part of the equation when it comes to fighting free radicals and oxidative stress, which are a large percentage of the equation when it comes to developing diseases.

Yet, unlike vitamins and minerals, scientists have not found a way to mimic the effects of phytochemicals in pill form. Sure, we can take a multivitamin it makes up for vitamin and mineral deficiencies in our diets, but the same is not true of phytochemicals. When scientists have attempted to put these in a pill it has proven unsuccessful. Scientists believe this is because there are many bioactive phytochemicals in plant foods, which work synergistically together to improve our health. Therefore, when these phytochemicals are isolated they are no longer able to work in tandem. This means that if you want to receive the health benefits of phytochemicals you must consume a varied diet full of a variety of plant matter.

The Ethical and Moral Choice

The benefits of choosing vegan go beyond the health and weight loss possibilities. In fact, by choosing the vegan diet you can make one of the greatest beneficial impacts on the environment as well as choosing to forgo the abusive animal-product industry.

While most people never think about where their animal-based products originated, the truth is that these products do a great deal of harm to animals. Even if you don't disagree with eating humanely-sourced animal products, the truth is that today's modern animal farming is anything but humane. While chickens, turkeys, pigs, cows, and other animals have the same emotions as pet dogs and cats, people often don't consider this when eating meat. While you would never consider eating a dog, most people don't think twice about eating a pig. The sad reality is that while these animals feel the same emotions as pets, they are often subjected to pain, grief, depression, and fear throughout their short lives. They are forced to live in small dirty environments, fed poorly, beaten by their handlers," and have their friends and family taken away. It is simply inhumane to put these animals through so much trauma.

This abuse inflicted on animals is not only in the meat industry but also in the egg and dairy industries, as well. People believe that these options must be more humane, after all, it doesn't involve eating the meat of the animal. Sadly, this is not true. After all, yearly millions of calves and cows are killed in the pursuit of producing dairy and billions of chickens and chicks in the development of eggs.

While chickens have been domesticated and altered at a genetic level to produce eggs nearly daily, prior to domestication chickens would only lay one or two dozen eggs a year. The difference in this number is staggering and leads chickens to experience chronic pain, reproductive disorders, and early death. As if that didn't make life miserable enough for the poor birds, their living conditions are also terrible. Over ninety-five percent of the chickens raised for the production of eggs are forced to live out their days in cages too small for their bodies, preventing them from so much as stretching their wings while seated.

Even so-called "free-range" and "cage-free" produced eggs still place chickens in dangerous living environments. These chickens are forced en masse to live in giant warehouses as if they were sardines in a can. The thousands of chickens can hardly move, and therefore have their beaks terribly and painfully removed to prevent them from anxiously pecking. Lastly, even if people raise chickens inhumane conditions in their backyards, the chicken still comes from terrible hatcheries. These hatcheries kill six billion make chicks yearly, both by suffocation and grinding them up while still alive. This is reprehensible and a large reason why vegans refuse to eat eggs.

Like the egg industry, the dairy industry causes an unimaginable amount of suffering. Just like humans and other mammals, cows only produce milk when needed to feed their young. Therefore, dairy farmers permanently separate a mother cow from her young within hours of their birth, all in order to steal her milk to bottle and sell. The female calves then grow up in agonizing conditions, without their mother, alone and isolated. On the other hand, the male calves are soon thereafter slaughtered to be sold as cheap beef. Once the mother cows are no longer useful, unable to produce the amount of milk demanded of them, then they too are killed.

There is more food on earth than ever before. In fact, there is so much food that we have enough to keep ten billion people well-fed. Yet, there are only seven billion people on the earth, eighty-two percent of these people are going hungry and malnourished. While classism and other factors play into this problem, one of the big factors that cause world hunger is the demand for animal-based products. This is due to the diet of the animals bred for the meat industry, which are fed half of all the grain grown worldwide. This grain, which could be fed to starving individuals, is used to fatten up animals lined up for slaughter. Many of these animals are not even grown in the Western world. Instead, they are grown overseas in impoverished and malnourished nations before being shipped to America and other first-world countries.

World hunger does not only occur overseas in impoverished nations but also locally. Your next-door neighbor may be unable to afford eating breakfast in the morning. The kids at your nearby school may only eat a single meal a day. Yet, while we have enough grains growing in America to feed eight-hundred million people, seventy percent of it is used in the raising of livestock.

Not only does the livestock industry waste grains, but it also wastes water. While some people never think about their carbon footprint when it comes to water consumption, it is important to consider. If you choose to go vegan you can save over seven-hundred thousand gallons of water yearly. Every single person who goes vegan makes a huge impact on the world around them.

Finally, the animal industry greatly increases pollution, worsening climate change. We all know that transportation contributes greatly to this pollution, but many are surprised to learn that for each calorie of typical feedlot beef it costs forty calories worth of fossil fuels. On the other hand, plant-based proteins only cost 2.2 calories of fossil fuels for each calorie of protein. The result is that eating a one-pound hamburger costs a shocking seventy-five kilograms of CO_2 emissions, which is the same amount of emissions produced when driving a car (at an average of three kilograms of CO_2 emissions daily) for three weeks.

These carbon emissions are damaging the planet and causing a mass extinction event amount many of the animal species that inhabit it. In fact, it is possible that we could have an ocean free of fish as early as 2048. If we want to take care of our homes and the next generation then we must take care of the earth and the animals which live here.

As you can see, there are many reasons to choose a vegan lifestyle. As you will see in the following chapter, the ketogenic diet also has many benefits. When you choose to combine these two lifestyles you are making a choice for a healthier life, better ethics, and a safer planet.

Chapter 2:

Keto 101

The ketogenic diet has been around for a century, originally developed to help people with epilepsy and other neurological disorders. However, the knowledge surrounding this diet has come and gone throughout that time due to a variety of circumstances. First, it was popular as the only way in which to reduce seizures, then it reduced in popularity due to the development of anticonvulsant medication. However, it again was on the rise when it was found that not everyone responded to drug treatment, some only saw results with the ketogenic diet. Most recently, the ketogenic diet has gained widespread recognition for its weight loss and other health benefits. Gone are the days when the ketogenic diet was only used for those with seizures. We now know it boosts metabolism, increases weight loss, and prevents or treats many of the most common diseases plaguing the world.

The Health Benefits of Keto

Before we look into how the ketogenic diet works at a fundamental and biological level, let's have a few of its many health benefits. As the anticonvulsant properties of the lifestyle are already well-known and researched, we will instead look at non-epileptic conditions which can be improved by the adaption of this method.

Weight Loss:
With many fads and crash diets, people yo-yo between one plan to the next, initially losing weight quickly, only for it to gradually come back. The result is that a person who yo-yo between one crash diets to the next may initially lose five or twenty pounds on a diet, only to continuously put on

more weight than they are losing. By the end of a year of doing this dieting, they can be sixty pounds heavier than when they began. Does this sound familiar? Sadly, it is all too common in modern society with magazines and articles selling one unhealthy crash diet after the next. Thankfully, there is another way. The ketogenic diet may be popular, but it is not a mere fad here one day and gone the next. Instead, this diet has withstood a century of use in the treatment of diseases. Unlike the crash diets which deprive your body of important calories and nutrients, the ketogenic lifestyle allows you to lose weight while eating your favorite foods. Can you enjoy avocados, almond butter, and chocolate? Certainly! While nobody should ever be shamed for their weight, and there is nothing wrong with being fat, it is true that having a high degree of body fat greatly increases the risk of disease and early mortality. Thankfully, you can lose weight while avoiding fad and crash diets with the vegan ketogenic lifestyle.

Unlike those other diets, the ketogenic lifestyle is different on a fundamental level. It is able to manage your insulin and blood sugar, which then reduce hunger cravings by preventing blood sugar highs and crashes. Therefore, you only have to eat when it is truly what your body needs, rather than listening to baseless hunger cravings.

When on a regular diet a person is constantly burning carbs within their body, which prevents them from using the fats they have eaten or stored as body fat. This causes gradual weight gain that could otherwise be prevented. However, when you are on a low-carb diet you are no longer burning these carbs, which allows your body to prioritize the burning of fats. This thereby boosts your metabolism and burns both dietary fats and body fat.

While most people come to the ketogenic diet looking to lose weight, it is possible that you can tailor it to gain weight if you are malnourished or underweight. There are many people who struggle to put weight on, which is just as unhealthy as being overweight. But, if you eat a vegan ketogenic diet with a high-calorie count you can slowly and gradually put on weight more easily than is otherwise possible, as there are many healthy high-fat and high-caloric foods you can enjoy. The specific amount of calories you need to eat in order to gain weight in a healthy manner will vary from person to person, so ask your doctor what your body requires.

Reduced the Risk of Heart Disease:
It is well-known that high cholesterol is the leading cause of heart disease. Yet, many Americans continue to eat foods that only increase the number of bad cholesterol while reducing the number of good cholesterol within their bodies. Yet, not only has the vegan diet been shown to drastically reduce cholesterol, so too has the ketogenic lifestyle.

There have now been many studies on the ketogenic diet and its effects on cholesterol and heart disease. Time and again these studies have found that the ketogenic diet only lowers bad cholesterol while increasing the body's natural good cholesterol. This is important, as good cholesterol is vital in managing hormones, increasing nutrient absorption, improving digestion, and removing the dangerous cholesterol from the body.

One of the studies on the ketogenic diet was conducted with the help of over sixty patients who were classified as "obese" and had high cholesterol numbers. After the individuals were placed on a ketogenic diet the researchers found that the participants lost weight, increased the number of good cholesterol, decreased blood glucose triglycerides, and lowered the overall number of bad cholesterol. The improvement was so significant that the researchers concluded the study to be a major success and that the ketogenic diet is a reliable and safe treatment option for those with heart disease and high cholesterol.

Treat Poly-cystic Ovary Syndrome:
Known to cause decreased fertility, irregular menstruation, insulin resistance, body hair growth, hyperinsulinemia, and weight gain, poly-cystic ovary syndrome (PCOS) is incredibly difficult to treat. In fact, there is still left to be learned about this disorder.

However, it has been found that the ketogenic diet can help a large portion of the people with this widespread endocrine disorder. In one study on the treatment of this disorder with the ketogenic diet, it was found that after being on the plan for twenty-four weeks (about six months) people improved drastically. Overall, there was an average reduction in fasting insulin by fifty-four percent, a thirty-six percent decrease in free testosterone, weight loss by twelve percent, and two of the people who had previously been infertile were even able to conceive.

Manage Alzheimer's Disease:

The occurrence of Alzheimer's disease and deaths caused by it have steadily increased over the past several decades, making it now the sixth leading cause of death in America. In fact, people usually only survive for four to eight years post diagnosis. The time period between diagnosis and death is not an easy one, as a person slowly loses their memories of their life and loved ones, meanwhile their family and friends have to watch them slip away.

Thankfully, recent studies have shown the ketogenic diet to be an exciting opportunity in Alzheimer's research and management. The reason that the ketogenic diet is such a powerful tool in Alzheimer's treatment is due to the biological core of how the lifestyle works. Put simply, the human brain with Alzheimer's disease develops insulin resistance. When this occurs, the neurons are no longer able to be fueled by glucose and carbohydrates effectively, causing the neurons to soon starve and become malnourished. Sadly, these neurons are unable to be fueled with either fat or protein. However, there is a fourth option: ketones. When you begin the ketogenic diet your body will convert protein and fats into both glucose and ketones. The glucose will be used for a few cells that need it, but many of these cells can also use ketones. Since ketones are a more effective form of fuel your brain will begin to fuel the neurons with ketones, which it is able to absorb despite insulin resistance. This helps to stop the starvation of your neurons, giving them a healthy and effective fuel source. Not only that but since the ketogenic diet treats insulin resistance it may also be able to treat the problem at its source.

With the addition of ketones people with Alzheimer's disease have been able to improve their memory and brain function, better respond to social situations and activities, walk better with less risk of injuries, and experienced fewer tremors allowing them to better complete daily tasks.

The ketogenic diet is a pioneering method in the treatment of Alzheimer's disease, and will hopefully help researchers find an answer to reducing the number of individuals affected in the near future.

Prevent or Treat Cancer:

We all know how devastating and deadly cancer is, yet, after searching for years we are still without a cure. While the cure for cancer is still out of sight, it has been found that the ketogenic diet can decrease your risk of developing this disease and improve treatment.

This is because cancer and tumor cells feed of glucose, which originates in carbohydrates. But, when you severely limit the consumption of carbs then the tumor cells are forced to starve a shrink, meanwhile, your body's natural cells are being fueled off of fat, protein, and ketones.

Studies have found that both cancerous and non-cancerous tumors can be reduced in size simply by enjoying a ketogenic diet. However, if the person once again begins to eat carbohydrates in the future, resupplying the tumor cells with glucose to feed on, the tumor will most likely once again grow in size. Therefore, the best course of action is a long-term ketogenic diet to continuously shrink the tumor. Even if a person needs to use surgery and chemotherapy to remove cancer from their bodies, by first shrinking the tumor size with the ketogenic diet it can greatly increase their chances for success.

Lastly, studies have found that not only is the ketogenic diet helpful in shrinking tumors, but it can also increase the effectiveness of chemotherapy while reducing the number of negative side effects experienced.

How Ketosis Works

The way the ketogenic diet works is through the ketosis process, which by definition is when your body contains very few carbohydrates and therefore begins to produce ketones as an alternative fuel source. This is a superior type of fuel, which especially helps the mitochondrial cells within our bodies.

There are thirty-seven trillion cells within the human body. Of these, about ninety percent are mitochondrial cells. The mitochondria within these cells are their powerhouse, which is able to use any of the fuel sources. This is the reason why a few cells in the body require glucose for fuel, but most are able to survive and thrive with any of the four fuel types (protein, fat, carbohydrates, and ketones.) The mitochondrial cells are imperative for overall health, since they convert ninety percent of the fuel we consume into energy, produce imperative biochemical reactions, recycle damaged cells into healthy cells, and remove damaging oxidants and toxins.

When using sources of fuel, ketones may be the best choice, but the mitochondrial cells naturally prioritize glucose. This is because the body can only hold two-thousand calories worth of carbohydrates at any given time. Any extra carbohydrates you consume before burning the calories off must be converted into fatty acids and stored as body fats. The body wants to avoid having to go the extra step of converting glucose into fatty acids, therefore it tries to prevent this by always burning glucose before other fuels. Not only that, but glucose is also a quicker source of fuel. While proteins and fats may take an hour or two to utilize, the body first must be in ketosis to produce ketones, it can instead utilize and burn glucose almost instantly after digestion. This allows quick energy whether you are running a marathon or completing your math finals.

Yet, while glucose may be a quick energy source it is not an effective fuel. In fact, out of the three dietary fuel sources (carbohydrates, fats, and protein), the only one the human body does not require us to consume is glucose. Yet, there is about ten percent of our cells which are not mitochondrial cells and require glucose to survive, but this is accounted for on a low-carbohydrate diet. How is that? It is known as the process of gluconeogenesis when the body converts protein (amino acids) into the amount of glucose the non-mitochondrial cells require. The gluconeogenesis process produces just the amount of glucose we need, without too little or too much.

While the human body does not require the consumption of glucose, it does need fat and protein to survive. There are types of protein (amino acids) and fat (fatty acids) which the body requires but is unable to create on its own. But, on the ketogenic diet, this vital amino and fatty acids are provided at a much better rate. These fuel sources are able to be used seamlessly for our mitochondrial cell and to be transmuted into both any needed glucose and ketones.

Ketones can be further increased with the consumption of medium-chain triglycerides, which is frequently found in coconut oil. These are a type of fat molecule that is shorter than most. Since medium-chain triglycerides digest more quickly than long-chain triglycerides they can be quickly and effectively used as fuel either as-is or once transmuted into ketones.

After you have been on a low-carb diet for a couple of days or up to a week you will enter the state of ketosis. Ketosis can be entered whenever your body is out of glucose to use as fuel such as when you are on the ketogenic diet, are fasting, or when you consume a large number of medium-chain triglycerides. The ketosis process is when your body begins to produce ketones. It does this by transmuting fatty acids into ketones, in the process it creates three types, known as acetone, acetoacetate, and beta-hydroxybutyrate.

There are many benefits to producing ketones. They are a more effective fuel source, lessen insulin resistance, increase weight loss, and they decrease the amount of protein that must be converted into glucose through gluconeogenesis. This is because while fat and protein are unable to fuel the ten percent of non-mitochondrial cells in the body (such as those in the brain,) ketones have the ability to pass through the blood-brain barrier and fuel most of these cells. Overall, when you are in ketosis your body has to use the gluconeogenesis process five times less than it otherwise would.

Some other benefits of the ketosis process and ketone bodies include:

- Ketones are a cleaner source of fuel than glucose. While glucose causes oxidants to form in the cells (such as in the brain,) ketones are just as fast-acting but without the byproduct of damaging oxidants. This is largely why the ketogenic diet is so powerful in treating conditions such as epilepsy and Alzheimer's disease because oxidants are known to cause disease. By not only preventing the formation of oxidants but also using ketones which remove these toxins from the body we are able to benefit our health at a cellular level.

- While a portion of the brain requires the gluconeogenesis process to convert protein into glucose for a fuel source, the remaining seventy-five percent of the brain and thrive with ketones as the sole fuel source.

- Oxygen is required in order to use the four fuel sources, which increases mental fatigue and the rate at which the brain ages. While glucose requires a large amount of oxygen, ketones only require a minimal amount, thereby increasing brain clarity and health.

- After a period of time of being in ketosis, your body will begin to produce more mitochondrial cells within the brain, meaning that more of your cells will be able to make use of any of the fuel sources.

- Inflammation is an important part of the immune system, butt in excess inflammation can cause more harm than good. In fact, people who have chronically high inflammation are more likely to die young. Thankfully, ketones have been shown to reduce inflammation through the entire body, including in the brain.

- Most of the brain's neurons are formed prior to birth, which is why it is so detrimental when neurological and neurodegenerative diseases cause harm to these neurons. Thankfully, ketones have been shown to replace a portion of damaged neurons with younger and healthier ones.

- Glutamate is an important nutrient for many of the body's basic function. However, an increase in glutamate can cause multiple sclerosis, Parkinson's disease, Alzheimer's disease, and Lou Gehrig's disease. Thankfully, ketones are able to keep glutamate balanced to a healthy level, both to help our normal functioning and to prevent these degenerative diseases.

Chapter 3:

Combining the Vegan and Ketogenic Lifestyles

Both the vegan and ketogenic diets are quite different from the average American diet. This is especially true when the two are combined into one healthy lifestyle. However, just because they are different from what you are used to doesn't mean it has to be difficult, confusing, or unsatisfying. On the contrary, you can follow a simple step by step process to adopt the vegan ketogenic life and enjoy satisfying food to its fullest, happy to know that the same food you enjoy can also benefit your health.

Most people don't think that vegan and ketogenic diets can go hand-in-hand. When they think keto they consider cheese, eggs, butter, and meat. Not only that, but you are unable to consume high-carb grains and legumes. Yet, combining the two into one is much easier than people first believe, all it takes is a little knowledge.

When you pair the vegan and ketogenic lifestyles together you can experience weight loss, health benefits, and satisfaction like never before. In this chapter, you will learn how to do just that, combining the two together in the simplest method. However, feel free to adjust your diet to your own taste. Maybe you feel like you want to remove grains or meats more quickly than other people, or perhaps you feel the need to slow down and remove these non-vegan and high-carb foods more slowly. Whatever you need, listen to your body and take the lifestyle one step at a time. Remember, this is not a journey of a single day, rather one you hope to continue to make day after day. Allow yourself to take the time you need to make the change easily and healthfully, in a way that causes you little to no stress.

If you have ever been either vegan or ketogenic in the past and didn't find you lost weight, don't give up hope. When these two lifestyles are combined into one it has many more benefits, including accelerated weight maintenance. Once you begin the vegan ketogenic diet, give yourself a full two months on the diet (after removing the non-vegan and high-carb foods) before deciding how it is going for you. Some people will judge that the lifestyle is too hard or makes them too fatigued during the first month. However, you cannot accurately tell at this point because your body and mind are still adjusting. If you give yourself a full two months eating a vegan ketogenic diet I am sure you will adjust in mind and body, experiencing increased weight loss, a boost in energy, better health, and a clearer mind.

When beginning your vegan and ketogenic lifestyle you want to make changes in steps, rather than all at once. Of course, there is the occasional person who finds it easier to make all the changes overnight and adjust over time. However, for most people, it is easier and less frustrating to make changes in small steps until they gradually work up to being completely vegan and keto. Take whichever method works best for you, but don't feel as if you have to jump right in. It is perfectly normal and okay to take your time. It is better to proceed in a manner that will help you maintain the diet long-term than diving in head-first.

Step One: Remove Junk Food

It is best to begin by removing junk foods. At this stage, you may still eat meat, dairy, whole grains, starchy vegetables, and other non-vegan and high-carb ingredients. However, you want to remove all food that would generally be classified as "junk." This means that you want to avoid fried, sugar-laden, and heavily processed foods. For instance, while you might still be eating cheese, you want to avoid Velveeta. You may still consume fruits and honey, but you want to avoid sodas (both regular and "diet") and candies. You may eat homemade pizza, but avoid takeout or frozen pizza which are heavily processed. While you can prepare homemade oven-baked French fries it is important to avoid fried or pre-prepared frozen fries.

In short, it is easy to know which foods are junk foods. Look at the label and avoid anything with sugar, high-fructose corn syrup, artificial sweeteners, excessive sodium, hydrogenated oils, trans fats, fried ingredients, or a number of preservatives and additives.

This first step can either be undertaken quickly or slowly. Some people choose to remove all junk food from their diet immediately, and it takes them a week or two to adjust. However, other people choose to slowly remove these ingredients from their diet over the period of a week or two. This does this by first removing one guilty pleasure (such as soda) and a few days later removing another until their diet is completely free from junk food. Both options are valid, and it is best to choose whichever method works best for you.

Step Two: Replace Carbs
On the ketogenic diet, most people need to consume no more than twenty-five net carbohydrates a day. Although, some people who are highly active, such as weight trainers, may be able to maintain up to fifty net carbohydrates a day. Yet, this is only for people who practice multiple hours of highly intense exercise daily. Your goal should be to aim for twenty to twenty-five net carbs daily, otherwise, you will have trouble entering ketosis.

Now that you have removed junk food from your diet it is time to replace carb-heavy ingredients with low-carb alternatives. There are three ways in which you can follow this method:

1. The most common method is to immediately replace all carb-heavy ingredients with replacements overnight. This will result in your body using up its storage of glucose at a good pace. Most people will enter ketosis within a day or two unless they have insulin resistance in which case it may take up to a week.

2. Some people choose to slowly integrate low-carb ingredients into their diet while removing carb-heavy options over the period of a week or two. While this method is completely valid, it can prolong "keto flu" symptoms in which a person's body is attempting to adjust to the ketosis process. It is often easier to use the first method, in which you immediately make the switch all at once.

3. The hardest method will get you into ketosis the quickest. With this third and final method a person will practice an intermittent fast for twelve to twenty-four hours, and then once they again begin to eat will immediately avoid any high-carb foods in favor of their lower carb options. By starting with a fast a person will enter ketosis rapidly, allowing them to adjust to the ketogenic process more quickly. While this method is speedy, it can be highly difficult for many people to fast. Therefore, consider your own strengths, weaknesses, and medical conditions before deciding which of the three methods you will choose.

Examples of high-carb foods you should be avoided include grains, sweeteners including honey and maple, starchy vegetables such as potatoes, legumes, beans, milk, low-fat dairy options, dried fruits, and sugar-heavy fruits such as bananas.

There are a number of alternatives that you can use, such as low-starch vegetables, cauliflower "rice," konjaku noodles, homemade low-carb bread, and stevia leaf and erythritol for natural low-carb sweeteners.

Step Three: Go Plant-Based

If you are choosing the vegan lifestyle for ethical reasons you likely want to begin overnight, not wanting to eat more meat, eggs, and dairy. However, while overnight vegan can work for many people, not everyone is able to do it. Know that if you have to slowly work toward becoming vegan that is completely okay! After all, every step you take is an improvement, and before long you will be completely vegan.

To become vegan it is generally easiest to focus on one ingredient or meal at a time. For instance, if you eat a lot of eggs you may decide to start replacing the eggs in your diet with scrambled tofu and other egg replacements. Or, you might decide to change a complete meal, serving yourself a daily vegan lunch or breakfast. Either way, if you choose to take it one ingredient or one meal at a time, you will find yourself adjusting to the vegan lifestyle naturally. Before long you will be well-acquainted with low-carb vegan protein alternatives and find it natural to use these in place of animal-based ingredients in your daily life.

Try replacing animal-based products with tofu, tempeh, soy milk, coconut milk, almond milk, coconut oil, olive oil, avocado oil, nuts, and seeds.

There are many dishes you can make with these, it is not limited to vegan "egg" scrambles. You can make "bacon" with tempeh, chocolate milk with soy milk, "cheese" with cashews, pudding with chia seeds, spreadable "butter' with coconut oil, and much more! There are a variety of recipes for the vegan lifestyle that is low in carbs which you can fully enjoy.

Don't worry if it takes you one to three weeks to make the change. All you need to do is take steps toward your goal one day and one meal at a time.

Step Four: Health Foods

In the last and final step, you simply want to catch anything you missed in the previous steps. For instance, you might have some foods in your diet that are low-carb and don't classify as junk food, but aren't health foods, either. The most common culprit for this is fats. Try to replace all of the fats in your kitchen with healthy options, such as avocado, olive, and coconut oils along with nuts and seeds.

Analyze your diet and see if there are any ways you can increase the number of healthy foods in your day-to-day life, create a better balance of varied fruits and vegetables rather than eating the same varieties with every meal, and ensure that you are including enough plant-based proteins throughout your day.

Chapter 4:

Eating Well with Macro and Micro Nutrients

By now you full well know the importance of protein, fats, and carbohydrates, or as they are otherwise known: the macronutrients. However, these nutrients which make up the largest portion of your diet can some confusing when you are first beginning the ketogenic diet. Thankfully, with just a little knowledge you will understand how much of these nutrients you should eat to enter ketosis, lose weight, and gain health benefits.

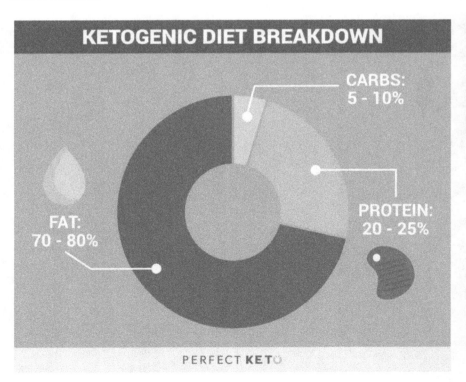

Not only are the macronutrients important, but so are micronutrients. These are the nutrients your body needs in smaller quantities but are still very much vital. This category includes both vitamins and minerals. You might be concerned if you can consume adequate micronutrients which vegan and keto, but, you will be happy to know it is entirely possible. All you need it to be prepared with the knowledge to ensure you are consuming all the nutrients you require and it will be simple.

In this chapter, you will learn everything you need to know about both macro and micronutrients so that you can arm yourself with the knowledge to have a successful and healthy vegan ketogenic diet.

Macronutrients

There are three macronutrients, which are protein, carbohydrates, and fats. While the human body is able to survive and thrive without any intake of carbohydrates, it relies on our diets for the addition of fats and proteins. Therefore, it is important to understand your macronutrients to ensure you get enough protein and fats while not consuming too many carbs.

Carbohydrates:

If you eat too many carbohydrates then you will be unable to maintain ketosis and will no longer produce ketones. This removes the benefits of the ketogenic diet, therefore, it is important that you maintain low levels of carb intake. Usually, between fifteen and thirty grams of net carbs are recommended per day, but most people aim for twenty-five net carbs. It is important to note that people who are highly active with strenuous exercises, such as weight lifters, may be able to consume up to fifty grams of net carbs and still maintain ketosis, but this is not common.

But, what are "net carbs"? The premise is simple. Fiber makes up a certain percentage of various carbs, and that fiber is not digested. Instead, the fiber is used to benefit digestion, increase nutrient absorption, and remove cholesterol before being dumped from the body. Since the fiber does not affect your blood sugar or insulin it does not need to be counted in how many carbs you are eating. In order to calculate the net carbs you simply have to read the nutrition label of a product and remove the "fiber" portion from the "total carbs." For instance, if the fiber is five grams and the total carb count is fifteen grams, then the net carb count is only ten grams.

Not only do you remove fiber from the net carb calculation, but you can often also remove any carbs from sugar alcohols. These are a type of fermented natural sugars that are non-alcoholic and generally not processed by the body. Just as fiber is dumped from the body, so too are sugar alcohols. Although, maltitol is an exception, which does affect blood sugar as it is partially absorbed. Thankfully, maltitol is now uncommon to use as it is known to cause digestive upset. The two most common types of sugar alcohols are erythritol and xylitol, both of which are perfectly fine to include in moderation on the vegan keto diet. When calculating net carbs, if you have either of these two sugar alcohols in an item you can remove the carbs from them from the total carb count. For instance, if a product has five total carbs and three carbs of erythritol, then the net carb count will only be two carbs.

Fats:

The main micronutrient that you will be consuming in large degree is fat. This can be fat from oils, avocados, olives, nuts, seeds, and other plant-based ingredients. However, it is important to be sure that you choose healthy versions of these fats, otherwise, you will not receive the health benefits of the vegan ketogenic diet. For this reason, you want to avoid oils that are void of nutritional content, such as corn oil, and replace them with healthy versions like avocado, olive, and coconut oils.

The specific amount of fat you will eat varies from person to person, just as every individual has their own ideal daily caloric intake. Since some people need to eat a great deal of food to maintain weight and others need to eat smaller portions in order to lose weight it can look quite different for the individual. Thankfully, you can easily know how much fat you should eat in a day with a keto calculator. These calculators, linked to in the Resources chapter, allow you to insert your personal information such as body weight, height, gender, activity level, and weight goals. Once the calculator has this information it is able to determine how many grams of carbs, fats, and proteins you should eat in a day to meet your goal for your specific body type. While one person may eat a thousand calories worth of fat a day, another might eat nearly two-thousand, it all depends on your individual calculations.

Proteins:

While it is important to ensure you are not eating too many carbohydrates and to consume the correct about of fats for your individual needs, it is imperative to eat your body's individual protein needs. Again, you will discover the number of grams you need to eat of protein when you get your keto macronutrient calculation.

Why is protein so important? If you don't consume enough you will begin to lose muscle mass and be unable to support your organ function, which relies upon the amino acids making up protein. Not only will that, but the gluconeogenesis process which transmutes amino acids into glucose to fuel neurons convert some of the protein you are eating into glucose. Yet, if you aren't eating enough protein then the gluconeogenesis process will be forced to break down your body's own muscles to use the amino acids found within them to fuel your brain. It is important to prevent this, so follow your keto calculations to ensure you are eating enough plant-based proteins.

Micronutrients

Micronutrients include vitamins and minerals, which are needed in a smaller amount than the macronutrients but are still just as vital for the body's normal functioning. For instance, if you don't consume enough of the vital electrolytes (sodium, magnesium, potassium, and calcium) then your nerves will be unable to communicate and your muscles will fail. Thankfully, these nutrients are found all throughout our diets, especially on the vegan ketogenic lifestyle. This allows you to ensure you can always find a source of vitamins and minerals. However, it is still possible to become deficient in micronutrients. In fact, over ninety-four percent of the population in America does not meet the minimal standards for at least one vitamin or mineral.

By understanding your body's needs for these nutrients you can ensure you eat adequate amounts to help your body thrive.

Sodium:

One of the four electrolytes, sodium is important for nerve communication and the functioning of our muscles. In fact, a deficiency in this mineral frequently causes people symptoms located in the heart and brain. Many people are worried about consuming too much sodium, but it is the opposite when you are on the vegan ketogenic diet. As you have removed processed junk foods you will no longer be consuming an overabundance of sodium. Not only will that but as you enter ketosis your body dump water weight, which takes the electrolytes with it.

It is important to refuel the electrolytes in your body as you lose weight, so be sure to salt your food. You may also need to add in a vegan and ketogenic sports drink option. You can buy a few options on the market or make your own. Keep in mind that if you are active you will especially need to ensure you are consuming enough electrolytes, as you lose them as you sweat.

Magnesium:

Many people develop magnesium deficiencies without being aware, yet this causes them to experience dizziness, fatigue, muscle spasms, and muscle cramps. As if that weren't bad enough, magnesium is vital for over three-hundred of the systems in our bodies', meaning that a deficiency in magnesium can be quite debilitating.

The daily recommended intake of this electrolyte is five-hundred milligrams for adults. Thankfully, you can easily get enough if you eat Swiss chard, pumpkin seeds, avocados, dark chocolate, nuts, and tofu. Magnesium can also be found in electrolyte drinks and certain supplements.

Potassium:

There are many high-potassium foods that are high in carbohydrates and therefore not keto-friendly, such as bananas. Yet, there are many other ways you can ensure you are eating enough of this vital electrolyte. The adult recommendation is forty-five hundred milligrams per day, which can easily be attained with the addition of avocados, kale, zucchini, pumpkin, eggplant, cucumbers, mushrooms, nuts, and tofu.

Try to avoid spinach for its potassium content, as spinach is high in oxalates. These oxalates prevent the absorption of vitamins and minerals, rendering it nearly useless. It is much better to stick with some of the other options.

Calcium:

Many people worry about consuming enough calcium on a vegan lifestyle. However, this electrolyte is found in many foods and is actually absorbed better from non-dairy sources. For instance, you can get calcium in broccoli, collard greens, bok choy, mustard greens, kale, sesame seeds, seaweed, and tofu. You can also consume fortified versions of soy, almond, and coconut milk.

Vitamin B12:

One of the most important vitamins to ensure you consume enough of when vegan is B12. This vitamin is easily neglected if you are unaware of what it can be found in and the importance of consuming an adequate enough. In fact, deficiencies in vitamin B12 are so severe that people can develop hallucinations, numbness in limbs, fatigue, tingling sensations, personality changes, blurred vision, memory loss, difficulty walking, sore tongues, and chronic pain. Yet, often these deficiencies get extreme before people are ever diagnosed, as people can go a year or even twenty years before their symptoms clearly illustrate the cause of the problem. Thankfully, there is an easy solution to this. You simply need to ensure you are eating enough vitamin B12, try taking a daily vegan multivitamin, and every six to twelve months have a checkup with your doctor. During your checkup, ask your doctor to run a vitamin and mineral panel. If you explain that you are vegan and want to ensure that you aren't developing any nutritional deficiencies they should understand and run the bloodwork for you. Choosing a vegan lifestyle isn't dangerous. After all, people of all lifestyles develop deficiencies, this is why ninety-four percent of America is deficient in one vitamin or another. However, because deficiencies are so prevalent it is important that we watch out for them and prevent them from occurring. Thankfully, if you do develop a deficiency it is often easily treated with supplements or simply increasing nutrient-dense foods in your everyday life.

B12 is the most difficult vitamin to get access to on the vegan diet, but this does not mean it is impossible. You can choose to use enriched soy, almond, or coconut milk. Another great option is enriched nutritional yeast. However, not all nutritional yeast is enriched, so make sure that yours is. One great brand is Bragg's.

Two tablespoons of Bragg's nutritional yeast contains eighty percent of your daily vitamin B12 needs, whereas one serving of Soy Dream Enriched Original Soymilk contains fifty percent of your B12 needs. That's not all, either! So Delicious is a popular brand of coconut milk, and their unsweetened original coconut milk contains fifty percent of your daily requirements.

As you can see, while there may not be an abundance of sources of vitamin B12, it is still easy to consume with just a couple servings of dairy-free milk or nutritional yeast. Better yet, nutritional yeast is often used as a cheese substitute, so it is incredibly tasty when added to meals!

Selenium:

A vital trace mineral, selenium is an antioxidant and supports the immune system. However, most foods rich in selenium are not vegan. Thankfully, there are other options! The single most abundant source of selenium is the humble Brazil nut, which contains five-hundred and fifty micro-grams in every single ounce of nuts! Yet, adults only need fifty micro-grams a day, which you can consume by eating only one-third of an ounce (9.5 grams) of

Brazil nuts. This is easy to chop up and add to meals, or simply enjoy it along with an afternoon snack. Be sure not to eat too many Brazil nuts though, as you can "overdose" in the mineral causing the condition selenosis.

Along with Brazil nuts, you can also consume mushrooms and chia seeds. Both button and shiitake mushrooms contain eighteen micro-grams for each half-cup serving, and each ounce of chia seeds contains fifteen micro-grams.

Vitamin K:

There are two types of vitamin K, which are K1 and K2. While it is easy to access vitamin K1 in vegan and ketogenic plant-based foods, it is harder to get K2. Actually, the only source of vegan vitamin K2 is fermented soybeans, known as natto in Japan.

Thankfully, you should be okay if you consume adequate levels of K1, as studies have found vegans who consume K1 do not have any adverse side effects. When consuming vitamin K (either K1 or K2) it is recommended for women to consume ninety micro-grams and men one-hundred and twenty micro-grams daily.

Vegan and ketogenic vitamin K1 sources include collard greens, kale, Swiss chard, broccoli, Brussels sprouts, parsley, cabbage, beet greens, soybean oil, and avocado.

While many Americans do not have access to natto or like the flavor, if you are willing to try to purchase some at an Asian market, online, or make your own you can get plenty of vitamin K2, other vitamins and minerals, and healthy probiotics by consuming these fermented beans. Eaten in moderation, natto can be enjoyed despite its carbohydrate count. Actually, since natto is made with soybeans it isn't overly high in carbs, a single quarter-cup serving only contains four net carbs.

Iodine:

Thirty percent of the worldwide population suffers from an iodine deficiency. This was worse in the past but improved when companies began to enrich table salt with iodine. However, now many people have switched to natural sea salts, which have many benefits but don't have the addition of the iodine. Therefore, it is important to ensure you are eating plenty of vegan and keto iodine-rich foods. This can be difficult, as there is no exact way to know how much iodine is within your food, as it depends on the soil the food was grown in. However, if you are worried you might not be consuming enough iodine naturally, then you can add seaweed to your diet. These sea vegetables are full of iodine, just avoid seaweed supplement tablets as these can cause an overdose in iodine.

Along with seaweed, you can ensure you are eating enough zucchini, green beans (which are low in carbs), spring greens, kale, watercress, and strawberries. While not nearly as high in iodine as seaweed, these ingredients tend to absorb more iodine from the soil they are grown in than other foods.

Chapter 5:

Intermittent Fasting for Weight Loss

Intermittent fasting, often shortened to "IF," is taking the modern world by storm. Why is it becoming so popular? Largely due to the increased knowledge surrounding the ketogenic diet. Since the keto dies utilizes long-lasting fuel sources of fat, protein, and ketones which keep you full and energized for hours on end, it becomes easier to fast. You can naturally go longer periods between meals, which not only increases weight loss but also benefits your health. Surprisingly to many people, intermittent fasting has even been shown in studies to increase lifespan and decrease the speed of aging!

Yet, despite the many benefits of intermittent fasting, many people have concerns. They worry that they will go hungry, deprive their body of nutrients, or that it is just another crash diet that damages your metabolism. Thankfully, none of these are true! In this chapter, we will ease any concerns you have on intermittent fasting, explain the process, and make it easy for you to implement in your daily life if you so choose. Going on the vegan ketogenic diet doesn't require intermittent fasting, but if you are attempting to lose weight it can be a wonderful way to boost your metabolism and fat loss.

With intermittent fasting you are not depriving yourself of nutrients, you are simply going longer between meals. This means that a person who is practicing fasting will consume the same number of calories as a person who isn't fasting. Both people may consume twelve-hundred calories a day, but while one person eats it between three or four meals, the person who is intermittent fasting eats those calories in only one or two meals. By going longer between meals your body will begin to burn its own fat as a fuel source, as it is naturally designed to do. During the past, humans would naturally practice intermittent fasting when they were working in the fields, hunting, or traveling. Yet, in modern times we almost always have quick and easy access to food. This causes us to consume smaller meals in rapid succession so that our bodies are always being forced to digest something. But, by stretching the time between meals you can give your body a break from digestion, allowing it to burn body fat and heal its own cells, overall improving your health.

Many studies have been conducted on intermittent fasting, and have found it to be much safer than dieting. Not only is it safe, but it is also beneficial for the human body. Along with being perfectly safe, there are multiple ways in which you can practice intermittent fasting. By having options you are able to choose what best works for you, ensuring that you are satisfied, energized, full, and happy.

However, while intermittent fasting has many health and weight loss benefits, it is best to wait until you have been fully in ketosis for a month or two before you begin practicing fasting. This is because when you first begin the ketogenic diet your body is not yet used to utilizing long-term fuel sources, which leads to hunger and fatigue until your body adjusts. Once you are well-acquainted with the process of ketosis you will be able to go longer periods without hunger or fatigue, as your body will be fully satisfied with the nutrients it has already been given. By this point, when you are well adjusted to ketosis, is the best time to practice intermittent fasting, as it often comes naturally. Since you feel less hungry you are likely to go longer periods without eating despite not actively attempting to fast. This natural fasting process signals that you are well into ketosis and able to easily practice intermittent fasting purposefully.

One of the easiest and simplest ways in which you begin practicing intermittent fasting is by skipping meals. This method of fasting should be followed naturally. For instance, if you eat a large breakfast and find you are still not hungry at lunchtime, simply skip lunch. You can eat again at dinner or have a snack in the late afternoon. By doing this your body will become accustomed to intermittent fasting, which is possible due to the protein, fat, and ketones fueling your cells. You won't have blood sugar crashes or fatigue. You simply will feel full, satisfied, and energized. Once you do notice yourself having hunger pangs again allow yourself to eat, it is as simple as that.

Most people don't skip dinner, as then they might get hungry in the middle of the night. Instead, most people have success with either skipping breakfast or lunch. Say you eat dinner one night at 6 pm, and then skip breakfast the next day. When you eat lunch at noon that has given you a natural eighteen hour fast. And, just because you skipped lunch doesn't mean you will miss out on food or nutrients at other times, as you can enjoy especially large and calorie-dense meals when you are not fasting.

Remember, this type of fasting should be natural. Don't push yourself to begin fasting too soon after starting the ketosis process or before you are adjusted to fasting. Simply eat when you are hungry and don't eat when you're not. There is no need to eat because it is a meal time if you are not hungry, so simply allow yourself to skip it if you want. It is okay if you, later on, decide to eat before your next meal time, you can have a snack.

Another quick and easy fast to accomplish is the twelve-hour fast. With this fast, you simply go half of the day without eating and fit all of your meals in the other half. This is easy, as you can begin and end the fast whenever is most convenient. For instance, you might begin the fast at 7 pm after dinner, and break your fast at 7 am when it is time for breakfast. Many people naturally don't eat between dinner and breakfast, and since you will be sleeping this fast is easy to maintain and fits into a busy daily life. Feel free to experiment with this fast so that it works best with your daily life. You can either shorten it or lengthen it to your preference, and move it to the time of day or night that is easiest to maintain.

Known as the Lean-gains diet, a sixteen hour fast is another popular option. With this type, you fast for sixteen hours of the day and eat your meals in the eight remaining hours. This can look many ways, but it is common to begin the fast after dinner and stop it at lunchtime. For example, you might finish your dinner at 7 pm. If this is the case, then you will want to eat your next meal at 11 am.

This fast is beneficial, as the longer fast will allow your body to burn fatter and better heal its own cells. Many of us are walking around every day ignorant of the damage happening at a cellular and biological level. Yet, with longer periods of intermittent fasting, such as with the sixteen hours fast, you can allow your body the chance to rest from the task of digestion and instead focus on healing itself.

Of course, you can shorten this fast if sixteen hours is too difficult for you, never force yourself to go into a fast or continue a fast if you feel the need to eat. Eat whenever you feel the need! In fact, many women will shorten this fast to be fourteen hours instead of sixteen, as it can be easier on their body, especially if they already struggle with their menstrual health and fertility. It is important to keep in mind that long periods of fasting (such as sixteen or more hours) can alter a person's menstrual health cycle. For some people, this alteration is an improvement in health, and for others, it is not. It all depends on the individual person, so listen to your body and do what it needs.

You will find that it is easy to turn this fast into a habit. While some people only fast two or three times a week, other people may fast on a daily basis. They simply are not hungry in the mornings, so they naturally fast for fourteen, sixteen, or even eighteen hours. This regular fasting has many benefits, but it shouldn't be forced. Allow yourself to take small steps toward fasting, instead of diving head first into it.

It is important to remember that when you are between fasting periods you must eat all that you require. You will know how much fat and protein you need to eat from your keto macronutrient calculation, and it is also important to consume foods high in micronutrients, such as vegetables.

While fasts sixteen hours and shorter are the most common, some people go more extreme with their intermittent fasting and will last for up to a full day. While this is possible, it is important for people who practice longer and more extreme fasting to never have two fasting days back to back. For instance, you wouldn't want to do a fast longer than sixteen hours on both Wednesday and Thursday. Instead, have some space between the fasts, you might try them on Tuesday and Thursday instead. This allows you to fuel your body with nutrients after one fast and before another, ensuring you are provided with all the macro and micronutrients your body requires.

Take intermittent fasting one day at a time, listen to your body, and be kind to yourself. If you follow these rules, then you will be able to naturally follow intermittent fasting at a healthy rate while also consuming the amount of food you need.

Chapter 6:

Tools and Equipment

By planning and prepping your meals you will save time, energy, and even money! As if that weren't beneficial enough, it will also allow you to prepare healthier and more balanced meals, helping you to increase your overall health and weight loss. In this chapter, we will discuss the best tools and equipment that will help you succeed with meal planning and prepping. While all of these tools aren't necessary, they are certainly helpful! If you can afford to invest in these supplies it will definitely be worth it. But, on the other hand, if you are unable to afford to buy new supplies that are okay, as well. It may be a little more difficult and time-consuming, but you will still be able to successfully plan and prep your meals.

Cutting Boards:
While people well-experienced in the kitchen know that you can't get by without a good cutting board, a lot of people new to cooking, planning, and prepping have yet to discover this vital tool. Thankfully, if you don't already have a cutting board you can easily buy a decent plastic one online for $15 for a single large one, or $18 for a set of three of various sizes. Of course, the prices will vary depending on the brand, store, and time of year.
It is important to use a cutting board because if you try to cut on your countertop or a glass plate you will run into many problems. Firstly, a plate is not the right shape or size to chop produce safely, you might accidentally cut yourself instead. Then, the countertop is not sanitary enough. If you are preparing food on your countertop you will be spreading germs and bacteria while also damaging your countertop. Thankfully, a cutting board can solve all these problems. It can easily be thrown in the dishwasher to avoid spreading germs if the cutting board

wears out over the years it isn't a problem since they are inexpensive to replace, and as it is the right shape for chopping you are less likely to injure yourself.

When buying a cutting board stick with plastic. You want to avoid glass, which causes your knife to slip and leads to injuries. Wood and bamboo are overly porous and absorb bacteria, which is trapped even after being washed. Therefore, plastic is the most practical choice.

Decent Knives:

Don't make do with whatever cheap knives you have stored in the kitchen. You never want to chop your vegetables with a small steak knife. Instead, it is best to invest in a full chef's knife set which will contain the full range of blades you require for any type of dish. You can buy these sets for a variety of prices. Cheap ones (which are made poorly) often cost around $25. If you want a nice knife set without spending $85-$150 you will want to buy one of the mid-range options, which often cost $50. These knife sets will often contain six to twelve knives, with a variety of blade types to cut anything you might need in the kitchen.

Remember, having the right knife for the job is imperative to avoid injury.

Digital Scale:

Having a digital scale is important on the ketogenic diet. It doesn't take long to weigh your food, but by doing this you know exactly how much you are eating. This isn't so that you can restrict your food, rather it is to help you meet your target macronutrient ratio. For instance, if you weigh out your ingredients you can figure out exactly how many grams of protein you are eating. Don't worry, these scales are inexpensive, you can get a decent one for an average of $10 minimum.

Non-Stick Mats:

When cooking in the oven there are many cases that food might stick to your baking sheet. This does not only make it more difficult to clean dishes later on, but it can even ruin your dish. Imagine that you have achieved the perfect crispy crust on your tofu, only to have it stick to the pan and fall off. This will greatly reduce the flavor and texture of your tofu. Thankfully, you can prevent this tragedy by investing in non-stick silicone baking mats.

These mats have decreased in price over the last few years. While they started out costing $30-$50 for a set of two, you can now buy them online for only $9 for a set of two. These mats are great because they can be reused time and again with a simple wash. This is helpful for both the environment and your wallet, as you don't have to replace it time and again as is the case with parchment paper.

You can even place these silicone mats on a pan before placing prepared items on the pan and then placing it in the freezer. Once the food is fully frozen it will easily peel off of the silicone pan and you can place it in a container. This makes it easy to store food in the freezer for a later date.

Crock-Pot:

I highly encourage investing in a Crock-Pot, especially for people who are always on the go. With this device, you can easily prepare your meal ahead of time, and then on the day you plan to eat the dish simply place it in the Crock-Pot two to eight hours before you plan to eat, go about your day-to-day business, and you will have a meal ready when you get home. This makes it easy to always have a freshly cooked home cooked meal after work or errands, without much effort.

Electric Pressure Cooker:

Like a Crock-Pot an electric pressure cooker allows you to prepare a meal, go about your day, and then have a hot and freshly cooked meal when you are ready to come home. However, unlike a Crock-Pot, pressure cookers don't focus on slow cooking. Instead, these devices cook food under high pressure, allowing them to cook in one-quarter or one-third of the time it would otherwise take. For instance, you might be able to cook "roasted" vegetables in twelve minutes instead of forty-five. You can cook practically anything in the electric pressure cooker, which makes it doubly helpful. However, these devices are rather pricey, as they usually cost between $70-$100. But, if you can afford to invest in purchasing the device you will find that it will save you time, energy, and even money in the long-run.

Blender:

With a blender, you can easily and quickly make creamy soups, smooth sauces and gravies, fruit and vegetable smoothies, and much more! These can be incredibly helpful, as there are many dishes you are unable to make without them. The prices of blenders vary greatly, with the Vita-mix being the most expensive by far. Although, you can also purchase affordable options with the brands Ninja, Oster, and Kitchen-aid at the regular superstores. If you are especially tight on money you might even watch the thrift store, where you might be able to find a decent blender for a couple of dollars.

Vegetable Spiralizer:

With a vegetable spiralizer, you can quickly and easily create vegetable "noodles." The most common option is using zucchini, but it is possible to use other vegetables, as well. With these spiralizers, costing anywhere between $5 to $30 you can create yourself low-carb vegetable noodles for pasta dishes, soups, and more.

Food Processor:

Being both vegan and keto you will have to chop a lot of vegetables in your daily life. This takes both time and energy. But, you can get this time and energy back if you use a food processor instead of a knife. With this device, you can quickly and easily chop up nearly any vegetable to a variety of sizes and types. Whether you need the food shredded, diced, or chopped a food processor can do it with its variety of blades and settings. A food processor can turn ten minutes of chopping vegetables into only two minutes.

Food processors are especially helpful for people with disabilities that affect their arms, as it saves them from having to use a knife. An average food processor will cost about $30 to $40, with higher-range options available.

Glass and Plastic Containers:

When preparing food ahead of time it is vital that you have containers to store the food in. You want containers that can be stored both in the fridge and freezer, ideally with a locking lid to prevent spills and stacking the ability to save space. You will want a variety of sizes of containers, both small and large, to fit anything you have to store from small servings of sauce to giant containers of soup.

It can also be helpful to invest in glass canning jars. These are a wonderful way to store liquid foods such as sauces, gravies, condiments, stocks, soups, and stews. By using these jars you can save space in the fridge and prevent spills. Not only that but with glass, you don't have to worry about chemicals leaching out of plastic.

It can take time to adjust to meal planning and prepping, but with time and practice, you will fall in love with the method. This process will allow you to save yourself time in your daily life, give you pre-prepared meals when you are at your busiest, save you time on busy days, and much more! You will love the new energy and time you find once you begin preparing your meals in advance. Now that you have an idea of what tools and equipment you will need, let's have a look at some vegan keto ingredients that are helpful to have stocked in the fridge, pantry, and freezer.

Chapter 7:

Meal Planning and Prepping

Instead of going day-by-day wondering what you can eat at the next meal, wouldn't it be nice to already have a delicious meal planned and prepared? Instead of relying on fast food, takeout, and meals from the frozen aisle of your grocery store you can enjoy healthy, filling, and satisfying home-cooked meals. These meals will not only make life easier for you, but it will also increase your health and make it much easier to stick to the vegan ketogenic lifestyle.

Most of us have had times in our lives where we were so hungry we were desperate to eat. It didn't matter what we ate and whether or not it was healthy, we simply needed food and needed it now. When hunger pangs strike and you become weak it is incredibly difficult to cook a meal or even consider what it is possible to eat. All you are left with is the ability to grab whatever food is easiest, quickest, and placed in front of you. Too often, this results in people eating fast food, desserts, or other unhealthy dishes. While it may be satisfying in the present, in the future we come to regret the decision. Thankfully, life doesn't have to be this way. Instead, you can choose to plan and prepare meals ahead of time, so that whenever you are hungry you always have one of your favorite dishes on hand and ready to enjoy.

Having a routine and plan is well-known to help people better succeed, in fact, many studies have proven this to be true. If you have ever looked at successful people, whether it's a nutritionist, athlete, or even a business owner, you will see that they all have one thing in common: they make use of schedules and plans. By having a plan you can succeed, as you no longer have to consider from day-to-day what to do. You already know how to succeed, you have laid the groundwork, and all you have to do is follow through by enjoying your prepared meals. By knowing you have food ready in the fridge, freezer, oven, Crock-Pot, or electric pressure cooker you will not be tempted to eat food you know you shouldn't.

There are many other benefits of planning and preparing meals ahead of time, as well. For example, you will find it becomes easier to develop nutritionally balanced meals. It is all too easy to eat the same ingredients time and again, but by doing this we do not get the variety of nutrients we need. Therefore, when you plan ahead of time you can ensure you eat a healthy balance of different vegetables, seeds, fats, and more.

You may also be able to prevent yourself from overeating. After all, if we are hungry in the afternoon we are likely to get a snack. Yet, if you already have dinner plans and know you have something cooking in the Crock-Pot you are more likely to hold out and wait for dinner time. By knowing when and what you will eat you are less likely to overeat, allowing you to better lose weight and increasing the ease of intermittent fasting.

For people on a budget, planning ahead can help to save money. After all, fast food, frozen meals, and takeout cost a lot more than a home-cooked meal. When you don't have a plan you also tend to buy more food than you require, allowing it to rot in the fridge before being thrown out. Yet, if you plan ahead you will know exactly how many meals you need, what you are going to do with leftovers, and won't be spending money on expensive fast food. You can even choose to shop sales and bulk ingredients, saving you even more money! This is possible because when planning your meals at the beginning of the week you can look at the sale papers for your local stores, find what produce and other ingredients are on sale, and then plan your meals according to what ingredients are best priced.

Yet, what is the difference in meal planning and prepping? They may sound similar and frequently go hand-in-hand, but they are quite different. In a meal plan, you decide what you are going to eat for the week(s) or month and write out a shopping list for the needed ingredients. This plan gives you a strategy of what you need to accomplish while you are preparing your meals. On the other hand, prepping comes after planning and it involves the shopping process; washing, chopping, and storing produce; marinating tofu and tempeh; cooking meals ahead of time; storing prepared ingredients or meals in the fridge and freezer. You can either store meal components, such as prepared tofu and vegetables, or fully cooked meals ready to enjoy.

Effortlessly Meal Plan and Prep

To begin meal planning it is important to decide what you are going to eat. You can plan ahead a week, two weeks, or even a month at a time. Try writing out a list of your favorite meals, or look online for vegan ketogenic recipes that strike your fancy. After you have a list of meals you can assign them to different days of the week for your schedule. Remember to plan breakfast, lunch, dinner, and also the occasional snack. However, this doesn't mean that you have to have a different meal for each of these eating times. You can choose to enjoy a certain meal one day and then enjoy the leftovers again later in the week. Of course, if you are someone who doesn't like leftovers you can either choose to make only small servings of dishes or freeze the leftovers to enjoy another week.

It is best to save recipes you like as you find them. If you are using a cookbook use sticky plastic tabs to mark your favorite pages. When looking at recipes online you can either bookmark your favorite recipes or save them on a website such as Pinterest. Even digital books will allow you to add bookmarks to pages, making it easier to find your favorite recipes at a later date. By saving your favorite recipes you can easily access them again in the future, making the meal planning stage much quicker and simpler.

When you are planning your meals try to keep things simple. This is especially important when you first begin planning so that you don't become overwhelmed and have difficulties. This means it is easiest to plan quick meals that are simple to assemble, repeated meals with leftovers, and meals that can easily be reheated or stored in the fridge. You don't need to create elaborate three or four-course meals when instead you can enjoy a hearty stew, tofu, and veggie noodle stir fry, or spaghetti squash with marinara and vegan cheese.

Another benefit of planning ahead of time is that you can plan out your macronutrient ratio. This is important to keep in mind because you want to ensure that you don't have too many carbs in a single day and that you are eating enough protein. To plan this out you don't have to analyze the nutrient density of every recipe (which is possible with various calculators online), but it is a good idea to have a general idea. For instance, if you are eating squash for dinner you don't want to eat too many nuts, which also have a decent number of carbs despite being generally ketogenic-friendly. You can also ensure that you pair a protein ingredient into every single meal. If you have a general idea of what is low-carb and what is high-carb you can easily plan a ketogenic week with a pretty balanced macro ratio. Then, once it is time to eat you can simply weigh or measure your food, input the ingredients into a keto calculator app, and you will know exactly how many macros you have eaten.

After you have planned your meals you can begin to prepare them ahead of time. To do this it is important to have a shopping list of every ingredient you will need to buy. While you can use a regular shopping list, it is helpful to have one that has ingredients organized by food categories. For instance, produce is stored together, fats together, seeds and nuts together, and so on. By having like-items organized together you can grab everything you need at once, without having to zig-zag around the grocery store. This saves both time and energy.

Once you get home from the store it is time to put all the food away. But, you don't want to put it away in the same way that you bought it. Instead, try to prepare some of your ingredients ahead of time. You can do this by dicing, chopping, grating, and turning vegetables into noodles. This allows you to easily grab your now prepped vegetables out of either the fridge or freezer whenever you are ready. Similarly, you can go ahead and marinate tofu to give it the best flavor possible.

When cooking meals ahead of time it is best to multitask in order to save time. For instance, if you have tofu and vegetables roasting in the oven you can also have a stew in the electric pressure cooker or Crock-Pot and sauces or condiments cooking on the stove. This will allow you to spend less time in the kitchen, but you do have to be more careful to not overcook or burn food since you are multitasking. You don't have to cook all of your meals in advance, but if you cook a couple or a few aspects ahead of time it can greatly help when you are busy, tired, or hungry.

Once you have a meal or ingredients prepared it is time to store it. You may either want to store it in the fridge or freezer. Generally, vegan food will stay fresh in the fridge for four to five days. If you plan to store food for any longer than this, then it is best to use the freezer. You can store the food in glass and plastic containers, glass jars, and plastic zip bags. While you can store stew in a single large container, some foods are better frozen individually. For instance, if you have prepared diced onions you don't want them to be stuck in a big frozen clump in a container. Therefore, you can spread the diced onions out on a silicone lined baking sheet, place it in the freezer, and allow them to freeze on the sheet. This is known as flash freezing as it freezes quickly and allows food to not stick together. Once the onions are fully frozen remove the pan from the freezer and place the frozen diced onions in a container back in the freezer. This will keep the onions from sticking together, allowing them to thaw and cook more quickly and letting you to only remove a certain portion of the onions rather than the entire container.

You may also choose to freeze prepared meals in the same way in individual servings. For instance, if you made a stew that you want to eat for multiple meals, such as lunches to take to work, you can measure the soup out into individual silicone containers. Small silicone pans, such as muffin pans, work wonderfully for this. You simply scoop the stew into each individual muffin cup, freeze the stew, and once it is fully frozen you can remove the stew cups from the pan and place them in a plastic bag to remain in the freezer. When you are ready to eat you simply remove one serving and either allow it to thaw or reheat it immediately.

By planning and preparing meals ahead of time you will find your life greatly improves. It may be a change from what you are used to, but you will soon find that it is well worth the effort.

Chapter 8:

4-Week Menu Plan and Shopping Lists

In this chapter, we are going to go into detail on a four-week menu plan, along with a master shopping list. With this shopping list, you can keep it on hand and simply write out or highlight the specific ingredients you need each week. This makes it easy, helping you to not forget anything important to buy.

The four-week shopping list will not only provide you with your first month of meals on the vegan ketogenic diet, but it will also give your ideas for further meals in the future. Use this menu plan for inspiration and then create your own.

Week One

Week 1:	Sunday:
Breakfast:	Tofu Scramble with Avocado and Roasted Tomatoes
Lunch:	Stuffed Mushrooms with Swiss Chard and Walnuts
Dinner:	Roasted Eggplant with Miso Tofu
Week 1:	Monday:
Breakfast:	Lemon Chia Seed Pudding
Lunch:	Coconut Curry Stir-Fry

Dinner:	Veggie Burgers with Cheesy Cauliflower
Week 1:	**Tuesday:**
Breakfast:	Green Protein Smoothie
Lunch:	Faux Potato Soup
Dinner:	Zucchini Noodles with Marinara and Meatless Balls
Week 1:	**Wednesday:**
Breakfast:	Chocolate Faux Oatmeal
Lunch:	Stuffed Mushrooms with Swiss Chard and Walnuts
Dinner:	Mushroom Steaks with Avocado Chimichurri
Week 1:	**Thursday:**
Breakfast:	Breakfast Burritos with Tofu Scramble and Tempeh "Bacon"
Lunch:	Creamy Broccoli Soup
Dinner:	Roasted Eggplant with Miso Tofu
Week 1:	**Friday:**
Breakfast:	Chocolate Raspberry Chia Seed Pudding
Lunch:	Kale Salad with Tomatoes, Avocado, Walnuts, and

	Strawberries
Dinner:	Thai Shirataki Almond Butter Noodles
Week 1:	**Saturday:**
Breakfast:	Tofu Scramble with Avocado and Roasted Tomatoes
Lunch:	Hearty Kale Stew
Dinner:	Roasted Eggplant with Miso Tofu

Week Two

Week 2:	Sunday:
Breakfast:	Almond Flour Pancakes with Lakanto "Maple" Syrup
Lunch:	Tofu Buffalo Wings
Dinner:	Lettuce Wrapped Veggie Burgers
Week 2:	Monday:
Breakfast:	Tofu Scramble with Cauliflower Hash browns
Lunch:	Cabbage Stew
Dinner:	Stuffed Spaghetti Squash
Week 2:	Tuesday:
Breakfast:	Strawberry Lemon Protein Smoothie
Lunch:	Creamy Broccoli Soup
Dinner:	Zucchini Noodles with Vegan Cheese Sauce and Roasted Tofu
Week 2:	Wednesday:
Breakfast:	Breakfast Burritos with Tofu Scramble and Tempeh "Bacon"
Lunch:	Bean Sprout Stir-Fry

Dinner:	Marinated Tofu Sandwiches with Cole Slaw
Week 2:	**Thursday:**
Breakfast:	Almond Flour Muffins
Lunch:	BLT Collard Green Wraps with Roasted Tempeh
Dinner:	Cabbage Steaks with Roasted Tofu
Week 2:	**Friday:**
Breakfast:	Bullet Coffee with a Side of Roasted Veggies
Lunch:	Broccoli Slaw with Blueberries and Edamame
Dinner:	Taco Salad with Cauliflower Rice, Guacamole, Sofritas, and Salsa
Week 2:	**Saturday:**
Breakfast:	Lemon Poppy seed Pancakes
Lunch:	Hearty Kale Stew
Dinner:	Spaghetti Squash with Basil, Garlic, and Sundried Tomatoes

Week Three

Week 3:	Sunday:
Breakfast:	Chocolate Coconut and Almond Chia Seed Pudding
Lunch:	Faux Potato Soup
Dinner:	Marinated Tofu Sandwiches with Cole Slaw
Week 3:	**Monday:**
Breakfast:	Chocolate Faux Oatmeal
Lunch:	Bean Sprout Stir-Fry
Dinner:	Zucchini Noodles with Marinara and Meatless Balls
Week 3:	**Tuesday:**
Breakfast:	Tofu Scramble with Avocado and Roasted Tomatoes
Lunch:	Tofu Buffalo Wings
Dinner:	BLT Collard Green Wraps with Roasted Tempeh
Week 3:	**Wednesday:**
Breakfast:	Green Protein Smoothie
Lunch:	Broccoli Slaw with Blueberries and Edamame
Dinner:	Zucchini Noodles with Vegan Cheese Sauce and Roasted Tofu

Week 3:	Thursday:
Breakfast:	Breakfast Burritos with Tofu Scramble and Tempeh "Bacon"
Lunch:	Creamy Broccoli Soup
Dinner:	Lettuce Wrapped Veggie Burgers
Week 3:	Friday:
Breakfast:	Bullet Coffee with a Side of Roasted Veggies
Lunch:	Stuffed Mushrooms with Swiss Chard and Walnuts
Dinner:	Vegan Pizza
Week 3:	Saturday
Breakfast:	Lemon Chia Seed Pudding
Lunch:	Cabbage Stew
Dinner:	Roasted Eggplant with Miso Tofu

Week Four

Week 4:	Sunday:
Breakfast:	Chocolate Pancakes
Lunch:	Broccoli Slaw with Blueberries and Edamame
Dinner:	Smoked Tofu with Zucchini Noodles and Nutty Sauce
Week 4:	**Monday:**
Breakfast:	Tofu Scramble with Avocado and Roasted Tomatoes
Lunch:	Broccoli Slaw with Blueberries and Edamame
Dinner:	Taco Salad with Cauliflower Rice, Guacamole, Sofritas, and Salsa
Week 4:	**Tuesday:**
Breakfast:	Cauliflower Hash browns with Tofu Bites
Lunch:	Kale Pesto Shirataki Noodles
Dinner:	Spaghetti Squash with Basil, Garlic, and Sundried Tomatoes
Week 4:	**Wednesday:**
Breakfast:	Bullet Coffee with a Side of Roasted Veggies
Lunch:	Creamy Mushroom Soup

Dinner:	Veggie Burgers with Cheesy Cauliflower
Week 4:	**Thursday:**
Breakfast:	Chocolate Faux Oatmeal
Lunch:	Coconut Curry Stir-Fry
Dinner:	Sofritas Soft Tacos
Week 4:	**Friday:**
Breakfast:	Green Protein Smoothie
Lunch:	Barbeque Tofu Veggie Bowl
Dinner:	BLT Collard Green Wraps with Roasted Tempeh
Week 4:	**Saturday**
Breakfast:	Orange Poppy seed Muffins
Lunch:	Cabbage Stew
Dinner:	Zucchini Pesto Noodles

Try using this list of common vegan keto ingredients when meal planning and prepping. They will help you to more easily create your shopping list and understand what is and isn't approved for the vegan ketogenic diet. There is a wide range of ingredients to enjoy, so play around and find new favorites!

Vegetables and Fruits

Arugula	Green Beans
Artichokes	Jicama
Asparagus	Kale
Avocados	Lemons
Bamboo Shoots	Limes
Beet Greens	Lettuce
Blackberries	Mushrooms
Blueberries	Okra
Bok Choy	Olives
Broccoli	Onions
Broccoli Sprouts	Parsley
Broccolini	Peppers
Brussels Sprouts	Pumpkin
Cabbage	Purslane
Cabbage (Nappa)	Radicchio

Cauliflower	Radishes
Celery	Raspberries
Chard	Rhubarb
Cilantro	Spaghetti Squash
Collard Greens	Spinach
Cranberries	Strawberries
Cucumbers	Summer Squash
Gooseberries	Tomatoes
Daikon	Turnips
Dandelion Greens	Turnip greens
Eggplant	Watercress
Endive	Zucchini
Fennel	

Protein Sources

Almonds	Tahini
Chia Seeds	Sesame Seeds
Walnuts	Sunflower Seeds (or Butter)
Brazil Nuts	Pumpkin Seeds
Hazelnuts	Pili Nuts

Macadamia Nuts	Tofu
Pecans	Seitan
Golden Flax Seeds	Soy Curls
Poppy Seeds	

Pantry Ingredients

Avocado Oil	Soy Milk
Olive Oil	Almond Milk
Coconut Oil	Coconut flour
MCT Oil	Almond Flour
Macadamia Nut Oil	Monk fruit Sweetener
Walnut Oil	Himalayan Salt
Sesame Seed Oil	Monk fruit Sweetener (Lakanto)
Cocoa Butter	
Coconut Cream	Sweet Leaf drops
Greek Dressing (Primal Kitchen)	Electrolyte Powder (Ultima)
Balsamic Vinaigrette (Primal Kitchen)	Zevia soda
Shirataki/Konjac Noodles	Zevia Energy
Coconut Aminos Soy Sauce Replacement	Water Enhancer (Stu)
Mushroom Seasoning	Water Drops (Sweet Leaf)
	Maple Flavored Syrup

Bragg's Nutritional Yeast	(Lakanto)
Spices and Herbs	Orrington Farms Vegan Broth Base
Coconut Milk	Agar Agar Powder
	Cocoa Powder

Chapter 9:

Recipes

In this chapter, you will find many recipes that will help you get well on your way to enjoying the vegan ketogenic diet. Many of these recipes were mentioned in the four-week menu plan, allowing you to enjoy the many meals the vegan ketogenic lifestyle has to offer.

Aquafaba

While aquafaba is not a meal in itself, it is an important ingredient for many dishes on the vegan ketogenic diet. This is because aquafaba is a low-carb and vegan egg replacement. It is made with chickpeas, but you don't actually eat the chickpeas, just the liquid they are cooked in, meaning that you don't have to worry about the carb limit!

Of course, if you don't have time to make your own aquafaba you can drain a can of chickpeas into a bowl and reserve the liquid. This liquid that the chickpeas are in is the aquafaba, which you can use in many recipes. Although, it is better to make your own aquafaba due to the sodium content in canned food.

When using aquafaba as an egg replacement:

1 Egg white = 2 tablespoons

1 Egg, whole = 3 tablespoons

The Details:

The Number of Servings: 18

The Time Needed to Prepare: 5 minutes

The Time Required to Cook: 60 minutes

The Total Preparation/Cook Time: 65 minutes

Number of Calories in Individual Servings: 10

Protein Grams: 0

Fat Grams: 0

Total Carbohydrates Grams: 0

Net Carbohydrates Grams: 0

The Ingredients:

Chickpeas, dry – 1 cup

Water – 4 cups, plus 2 tablespoons

The Instructions:

4. Place the chickpeas in a bowl of water and allow them to soak overnight or for eight hours.

5. After the chickpeas are done cooking drain the water away rinse, the chickpeas, and place them in a pot. Add the water to the pot along with the chickpeas, cover the pot with a lid, and bring it to a boil.

6. Be careful and keep a close eye on the chickpeas, as they easily boil over. Once the chickpeas have come to a boil they will produce foam in the water. Use a slotted spoon and continuously skim off this foam until the water is clear. Discard the foam.

7. Decrease the heat of the chickpeas to low and allow them to simmer with the lid on until they become tender for about one hour.

8. Turn the heat off of the stove and allow the chickpeas to cool while remaining in the water. This step is important, as the water will continue to be infused with the proteins from the chickpeas, allowing it to make a good binding agent and egg replacer.

9. Once the water is cool remove the chickpeas from the liquid and

discard them or give them to someone who can utilize them (as they are not low-carb). Place the aquafaba in a jar and store it in the fridge using it as needed. Or, you can freeze it in small individual servings, so that you only ever have to thaw out as much as you need.

Almond Flour Pancakes

These pancakes are the perfect weekend treat, even better since there are multiple flavor options! Below the recipe, in the Notes section, you will find three flavor options so that you can always enjoy new and fresh pancakes. Don't feel like plain (but delicious) pancakes? That's fine, why not make chocolate, blueberry, or even lemon poppy seed? Kids and adults alike will love these for breakfast or dinner!

The Details:

The Number of Servings: 2

The Time Needed to Prepare: 5 minutes

The Time Required to Cook: 20 minutes

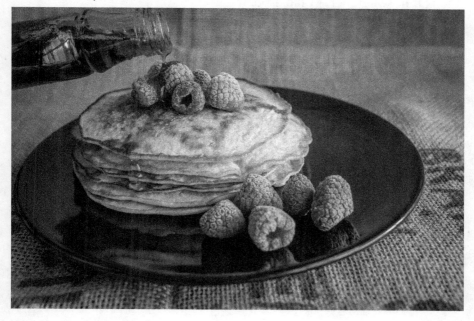

The Total Preparation/Cook Time: 25 minutes

Number of Calories in Individual Servings: 420

Protein Grams: 10

Fat Grams: 37

Total Carbohydrates Grams: 5

Net Carbohydrates Grams: 6

The Ingredients:

Almond Flour – 1 cup

Olive oil – 2 tablespoons

Sea salt - .25 teaspoon

Baking powder – 1 teaspoon

Vanilla extract – 1 teaspoon

Soy milk – 2 tablespoons

Monk fruit sweetener – 1 tablespoon

Aquafaba – 6 tablespoons

The Instructions:

- On the stove place a large metal skillet with non-stick coating and allow it to heat over a temperature of medium-low.

- Meanwhile, in a bowl whisk together the aquafaba, monk fruit sweetener, soy milk, vanilla extract, and olive oil. Once done, add in the almond flour, sea salt, and baking powder, stirring together until there are no clumps. However, be careful to not overmix the pancake batter, just mix it until done, otherwise they won't be fluffy.

- If using any of the optional mix-ins (below the recipe's directions) mix them into the batter at this point.

- Using butter or coconut oil grease the preheated skillet and pour the pancake batter into little disks, each pancake containing three to four tablespoons each. You can easily measure out the pancake batter using a .25 cup scoop to ensure they are all the same size.

- Allow the almond flour pancakes to cook until they begin to set up and bubbles begin to form, and then once they are sturdy use a spatula and gently flip them over. Each side should need to cook for about three to four minutes. However, watch the pancakes closely because if your stove is too hot the almonds can burn quickly.

- Remove the pancakes from the skillet once they are done cooking and repeat the process until all of the pancakes are cooked. You should be left with about six small to medium pancakes, perfect for two individuals. Enjoy the pancakes with fruit, sweetened coconut cream, or Lakanto's maple-flavored syrup.

Notes:

For Chocolate Pancakes:
Cocoa Powder – 1.5 tablespoons
Lily's Stevia-Sweetened Chocolate, chopped – 2 ounces

For Blueberry Pancakes:
Blueberries - .25 cup

For Lemon Poppy Seed Pancakes:
Lemon juice – 2 tablespoons in place of the soy milk
Lemon zest - .5 teaspoon
Poppy seeds – 2 teaspoons

Tofu Egg Scramble

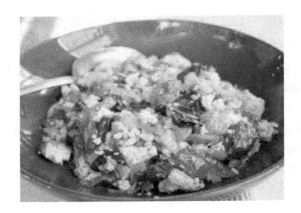

This tofu "egg" scramble is quick and easy to make, and people won't believe that it's not real eggs! Anyone will enjoy these alongside roasted tomatoes, avocados, tempeh "bacon," or other traditional breakfast options.

The Details:

The Number of Servings: 4

The Time Needed to Prepare: 5 minutes

The Time Required to Cook: 10 minutes

The Total Preparation/Cook Time: 15 minutes

Number of Calories in Individual Servings: 187

Protein Grams: 12

Fat Grams: 14

Total Carbohydrates Grams: 5

Net Carbohydrates Grams: 4

The Ingredients:

Tofu, extra firm – 16 ounces

Avocado oil – 1 tablespoon

Nutritional yeast – 2 tablespoons

Garlic powder – 1 teaspoon

Onion powder - .5 teaspoon

Black pepper - .25 teaspoon

Turmeric, ground – 1 teaspoon

Dijon mustard – 2 teaspoons

Soy milk - .33 cup

Sea salt - .75 teaspoon

The Instructions:

1. Use a fork to gently mash the tofu into medium to large chunks. You don't want to overly mash the tofu, instead try to get the chunks into the same size as scrambled egg chunks.

2. In a bowl whisk together the soy milk with the nutritional yeast and other seasonings until it is smooth.

3. Pour the avocado oil into a non-stick coated large skillet and allow it to heat over medium-high heat. Add in the tofu and panfry it in the oil until it is lightly browned, being careful to not break up the chunks too much with the spoon when stirring.

4. After the tofu has browned add in the sauce and gently fold it into the tofu. Continue to cook the tofu until it reaches your desired consistency, as the tofu will continue to absorb the sauce while it cooks. You can decide how dry you want it to be.

5. Serve the scrambled tofu alone, with vegetables, in soft tacos, and more.

Chia Seed Pudding

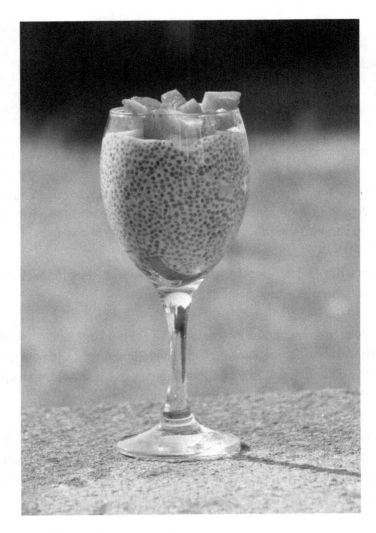

If you like tapioca pudding, you will love this easy and low-carb alternative! All you have to do is combine a handful of ingredients and allow them to chill in the refrigerator. Once cool you will have a delicious pudding. While this recipe makes a basic vanilla pudding, you can turn it into many different flavors! Look in the recipe's note from some flavor ideas.

The Details:

The Number of Servings: 3

The Time Needed to Prepare: 5 minutes

The Time Required to Cook: 0 minutes

The Total Preparation/Cook Time: 65 minutes

Number of Calories in Individual Servings: 366

Protein Grams: 5

Fat Grams: 36

Total Carbohydrates Grams: 10

Net Carbohydrates Grams: 6

The Ingredients:

Chia seeds - .5 cup

Coconut milk, full-fat, canned – 2 cups

Vanilla extract – 2 teaspoons

Erythritol/Stevia sweetener – 2 tablespoons

The Instructions:

1. Place all of the ingredients together in a bowl, container, or jar and mix them together well until there are no clumps of chia remaining.

2. Cover the container and place it in the fridge, stirring it once every fifteen to twenty minutes. After an hour the chia pudding should be ready. Serve immediately or store it in the fridge until ready to enjoy.

Notes:

- **Lemon Poppy Seed**
  Lemon juice – 2 tablespoons
  Lemon zest - .5 teaspoon
  Poppy seeds – 1 tablespoon

- **Chocolate Raspberry**
  Cocoa – 3 tablespoons
  Raspberries, gently mashed - .25 cup

- **Chocolate Coconut**
  Cocoa – 3 tablespoons
  Toasted coconut, unsweetened - .25 cup
  Almonds, toasted, chopped – 2 tablespoons

Chocolate Faux Oatmeal

These "oats" are made with low-carb and high protein seeds, which are full of nutrition. When you enjoy these faux oats you will be enabling yourself to feel energy and satisfaction all day long, as they stick with you and supply any nutrition you might need.

The Details:

The Number of Servings: 2

The Time Needed to Prepare: 2 minutes

The Time Required to Cook: 5 minutes

The Total Preparation/Cook Time: 7 minutes

Number of Calories in Individual Servings: 370

Protein Grams: 11

Fat Grams: 32

Total Carbohydrates Grams: 9

Net Carbohydrates Grams: 4

The Ingredients:

Golden flax seed, meal – 1 tablespoon

Hemp seeds, hulled - .25 cup

Chia seeds - .5 tablespoon

Erythritol/Stevia sweetener – 1 tablespoon

Sea salt – .25 teaspoon

Coconut milk, full-fat, canned – .5 cup, plus 1 tablespoon

Almond butter – 1 tablespoon

Lily's Stevia-Sweetened Chocolate Chips – 1 tablespoon

The Instructions:

1. Combine all of the ingredients except for the almond butter and chocolate chips together in a small saucepan. Place the prepared saucepan on your stove and allow it to heat over medium-high heat.

2. Stir the faux oats while they cook until they absorb the liquid and become hot, which should take about five minutes.

3. Remove the faux oats from the heat, stir in the almond butter and chocolate chips, and serve.

Tempeh Bacon

Just because you can't eat bacon on the vegan lifestyle doesn't mean you can't enjoy the flavor! Make this tempeh "bacon" to enjoy the classic favorite while still sticking to your diet.

The Details:

The Number of Servings: 3

The Time Needed to Prepare: 5 minutes

The Time Required to Cook: 15 minutes

The Total Preparation/Cook Time: 20 minutes

Number of Calories in Individual Servings: 162

Protein Grams: 8

Fat Grams: 13

Total Carbohydrates Grams: 4

Net Carbohydrates Grams: 4

The Ingredients:

Tempeh, sliced into thin strips – 4 ounces

Lakanto Maple-Flavored Syrup – 1 tablespoon

Sea salt -5 teaspoon

Water – 1 tablespoon

Tamari sauce – 2 tablespoons

Liquid smoke – 5 teaspoon

Garlic powder - 5 teaspoon

Black pepper, ground - .25 teaspoon

Olive oil – 2 tablespoons

The Instructions:

1. Pour the olive oil into a medium non-stick skillet over a temperature of medium heat and allow it to warm up. Add in the tempeh strips and cook each side until crispy and browned, about five minutes each.

2. Add the water, tamari sauce, liquid smoke, and seasonings into the skillet, stirring the ingredients together until the tempeh is evenly coated.

3. Allow the tempeh now coated in seasonings to brown for an additional two to three minutes before removing from the pan.

Creamy Broccoli Soup

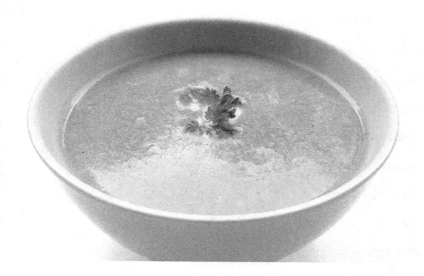

This soup is the perfect option for either lunch or dinner, as it can fill you right up. Enjoy this soup alone or with a grain-free vegan and keto bread and nut "cheese".

The Details:

The Number of Servings: 5

The Time Needed to Prepare: 3 minutes

The Time Required to Cook: 27 minutes

The Total Preparation/Cook Time: 30 minutes

Number of Calories in Individual Servings: 116

Protein Grams: 5

Fat Grams: 6

Total Carbohydrates Grams: 11

Net Carbohydrates Grams: 7

The Ingredients:

Broccoli, chopped – 6 cups

Garlic, minced – 5 cloves

Celery, chopped – 2 ribs

Sea salt – 1.5 teaspoons

Soy milk – 1 cup

Onion powder – 1 teaspoon

Vegetable broth – 3 cups

Olive oil – 2 tablespoons

Black pepper, ground - .5 teaspoon

The Instructions:

1. Place the celery and olive oil in a pot and allow it to cook for a few minutes, until becoming tender. You should have the temperature of the pot set to medium heat. Add in the minced garlic and seasonings, allowing them to cook together for an additional minute or two until the garlic becomes fragrant. Be sure to not burn the garlic.

2. Add the chopped garlic, soy milk, and broth to the stove, allowing the ingredients to simmer together for twenty minutes until the broccoli is tender.

3. Allow the broccoli soup to cool for a few minutes before carefully transferring it to a blender and pulsing until smooth. Be careful, because if the soup is still hot the pressure from the steam can add up and cause the lid to pop off. You can either blend the soup until completely smooth or leave it slightly chunky.

4. Serve the soup immediately or reheat it on the stove before serving.

Tofu Buffalo Wings

These Buffalo wings are amazing, and perfect for any wings lover! You can either enjoy them on their own or with your favorite vegan and keto Ranch dressing. Try these with the Primal Kitchen Ranch Dressing and you will fall in love!

The Details:

The Number of Servings: 5

The Time Needed to Prepare: 5 minutes

The Time Required to Cook: 10 minutes

The Total Preparation/Cook Time: 15 minutes

Number of Calories in Individual Servings: 238

Protein Grams: 8

Fat Grams: 22

Total Carbohydrates Grams: 2

Net Carbohydrates Grams: 2

The Ingredients:

Tofu, extra-firm – 16 ounces

Psyllium husk – 2 tablespoons

Garlic powder - .25 teaspoon

Sea salt - .4 teaspoon

Olive oil – 3 tablespoons

Vegan butter - .25 cup

Tamari sauce – 1 teaspoon

White vinegar – 1 tablespoon

Frank's Original Red Hot Sauce - .33 cup

Garlic powder - .25 teaspoon

The Instructions:

1. Place one-quarter of a teaspoon of garlic powder into a glass bowl along with the tamari sauce, vinegar, vegan butter, and Frank's Hot Sauce. Stir the ingredients together before melting them in the microwave. After the butter has melted whisk the ingredients until combined into a sauce and set aside.

2. Slice the tofu into medium-sized cubes, about half to one inch in size. Place the tofu cubes in a bowl and toss them with the remaining garlic powder, sea salt, and psyllium husk until the tofu is evenly coated. Be gentle so that you do not break the tofu cubes.

3. Place the olive oil in a large non-stick pan for frying and heat it over a temperature of medium-high. Add the tofu and allow it to fry on all sides until golden-brown and crispy, about a few minutes on each side.

4. Remove the tofu from the heat and place it in a heat-safe bowl, adding in the prepared buffalo sauce, tossing them together until the tofu has absorbed all of the sauce.

5. Serve the Buffalo wings alone or with vegan/keto Ranch dressing.

BLT Collard Green Wraps

These wraps are quick and easy to make, all you need to do is grab some produce out of the fridge along with some leftover tempeh bacon. Enjoy this alone or with a friend, either way, you are sure to love these wraps!

The Details:

The Number of Servings: 1

The Time Needed to Prepare: 5 minutes

The Time Required to Cook: 0 minutes

The Total Preparation/Cook Time: 5 minutes

Number of Calories in Individual Servings: 445

Protein Grams: 11

Fat Grams: 22

Total Carbohydrates Grams: 14

Net Carbohydrates Grams: 4

The Ingredients:

Collard green leaves, large – 2

Tempeh Bacon – 2 servings

Cucumber, sliced - .5 cup

Roma tomatoes, sliced – 1

Vegan mayonnaise – 2 tablespoons

The Instructions:

- Wash and dry the collard green leaves before using a knife to remove the stem. Once the stem is removed, lay the leaves out on a flat surface.

- Smear the top side of the leaves with the vegan mayonnaise, add in the tempeh bacon, cucumber, and Roma tomatoes. Wrap in the ends of the collard green leaves and then the sides, folding it like a burrito. Slice both wraps in half and serve.

Broccoli Slaw with Blueberries and Edamame

This slaw is delicious with a variety of textures and flavors, you will love the blueberries and edamame found within. Enjoy this dish on its own, or alongside another favorite meal.

The Details:

The Number of Servings: 4

The Time Needed to Prepare: 5 minutes

The Time Required to Cook: 0 minutes

The Total Preparation/Cook Time: 5 minutes

Number of Calories in Individual Servings: 92

Protein Grams: 5

Fat Grams: 4

Total Carbohydrates Grams: 11

Net Carbohydrates Grams: 7

The Ingredients:

Broccoli slaw mix – 12 ounces

Vegan mayonnaise – 2 tablespoons

Red onion, diced - .25 cup

Parsley, fresh, chopped – 1 tablespoon

Blueberries - .5 cup

Edamame - .5 cup

Sea salt – 1 teaspoon

Apple cider vinegar - .5 teaspoon

Erythritol/Stevia sweetener – .5 tablespoon

Lemon juice – 1 tablespoon

Black pepper, ground - .25 teaspoon

The Instructions:

1. Place the broccoli slaw, red onion, parsley, blueberries, and edamame together in a salad bowl and set it aside.

2. In a small bowl whisk together the vegan mayonnaise, erythritol sweetener, vinegar, lemon juice, and seasonings. Once fully combined pour this mixture over the slaw.

3. Using tongs toss together the broccoli slaw until it is well coated in the dressing and serve immediately.

Veggie Burgers

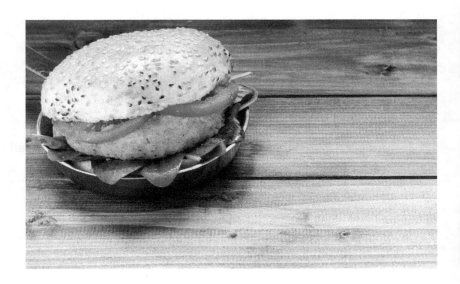

Whether you serve these burgers alone, in a vegan/keto bun, or with a side of roasted zucchini garlic fries, you will love them! Try them with your favorite toppings and you will soon have a new favorite burger.

The Details:

The Number of Servings: 4

The Time Needed to Prepare: 10 minutes

The Time Required to Cook: 55 minutes

The Total Preparation/Cook Time: 45 minutes

Number of Calories in Individual Servings: 123

Protein Grams: 5

Fat Grams: 6

Total Carbohydrates Grams: 13

Net Carbohydrates Grams: 6

The Ingredients:

Cauliflower rice – 10 ounces

Mushrooms, finely diced – 8 ounces

Onion, finely diced - .5 cup

Celery, finely diced - .5 cup

Garlic, minced – 2 cloves

Olive oil – 1 tablespoon

Tamari sauce – 1 teaspoon

Paprika, smoked - .25 teaspoon

Parsley, dried – 1 teaspoon

Cumin, ground – .25 teaspoon

Garlic powder - .25 teaspoon

Sea salt - .5 teaspoon

Chia seeds – 1 tablespoon

Golden flax meal - .25 cup

The Instructions:

1. Place the olive oil in a large pan over medium heat before adding in the garlic, celery, and onion. Allow the veggies to cook for two to three minutes until they begin to soften. Add in the cauliflower rice and mushrooms, continuing to cook and stir for ten to twelve minutes. You want to cook this until as much of the moisture is cooked out of the vegetables as possible. Remove the pan from the stove's burner.

2. Preheat your oven to the hot temperature of four-hundred degrees Fahrenheit.

3. Add the soy sauce and seasonings to the vegetable burger mixture, combining it well. Add in the chia seeds and flax seeds, combining them until combined. Set the mixture aside and let it cool down for five to ten minutes, which will allow it to thicken.

4. Line a large baking sheet with parchment paper (not a silicone mat). Once the vegetable mixture has cooled down divide it into four evenly sized patties. The mixture will be sticky but should come together easily. It is best to oil your hands to prevent the mixture from sticking.

5. If your vegetable mixture isn't sticking together well you may need to add one or two more tablespoons of flax seed meal and allow it to absorb for a few minutes before continuing to make the patties.

6. Place the pan of burgers into the center of a large kitchen oven that is preheated until they are browned and crispy, about thirty minutes. After removing the burgers from the oven allow them to cool for five minutes before serving.

Mushroom Steaks with Avocado Chimichurri

These mushrooms steaks are quick and easy to make, yet full of flavor from their marinade and the avocado chimichurri. These are delicious year-round, but the chimichurri makes them especially wonderful for a summer evening.

The Details:

The Number of Servings: 4

The Time Needed to Prepare: 15 minutes

The Time Required to Cook: 10 minutes

The Total Preparation/Cook Time: 25 minutes

Number of Calories in Individual Servings: 355

Protein Grams: 5

Fat Grams: 31

Total Carbohydrates Grams: 16

Net Carbohydrates Grams: 10

The Ingredients:

Portobello mushrooms stem removed, cleaned – 4

Olive oil - .25 cup

Balsamic vinegar - .33 cup

Black pepper, ground - .5 teaspoon

Cumin, ground - .5 teaspoon

Paprika, smoked - .25 teaspoon

Garlic, minced – 3 cloves

Tomato paste – .5 tablespoon

White vinegar - .5 tablespoon

Erythritol/Stevia sweetener - .5 teaspoon

Avocado, diced – 1

Garlic, minced – 3 cloves

Parsley, fresh, chopped – 1.5 cups

Red pepper flakes - .25 teaspoon

Shallot, minced – 1

Lemon juice – 3 tablespoons

Olive oil – 3 tablespoons

Sea salt – .5 teaspoon

The Instructions:

1. In a bowl whisk together the one-quarter cup of olive oil, three tablespoons of the garlic, black pepper, balsamic vinegar, cumin, paprika, tomato paste, white vinegar, and the sweetener.

2. Place the mushrooms in a shallow baking dish and top it with the marinade, using a pastry brush to cover all the crevices. Allow them to marinate for five minutes, flip the mushrooms over and brush them with the sauce, and allow them to marinate for an additional five minutes.

3. While the mushrooms marinate toss together the remaining garlic, parsley, remaining olive oil, red pepper flakes, shallow, sea salt, and lemon juice. Add in the avocado and toss to combine. Set the chimichurri aside.

4. Heat a large skillet to a temperature of the medium and then add in the mushrooms, allowing each side to sear and caramelize for two to three minutes.

5. Remove the mushrooms from the heat and top them off with the avocado chimichurri.

Sofritas

These sofritas are reminiscent of those served at a popular Mexican restaurant in America. But, instead of spending a fortune going out to eat you can easily and affordably make your own!

The Details:

The Number of Servings: 4

The Time Needed to Prepare: 5 minutes

The Time Required to Cook: 0 minutes

The Total Preparation/Cook Time: 5 minutes

Number of Calories in Individual Servings: 92

Protein Grams: 5

Fat Grams: 4

Total Carbohydrates Grams: 11

Net Carbohydrates Grams: 7

The Ingredients:

Tofu, extra firm – 16 ounces

Olive oil – 1 tablespoon

Cumin – 1 teaspoon

Garlic, minced – 2 cloves

Chipotle chiles – 2

Anchi chili powder – 1 teaspoon

Onion, diced - .5

Roma tomato, diced – 1

Oregano, dried - .5 teaspoon

Adobo sauce – 2 tablespoons

Sea salt - .5 teaspoon

Red wine vinegar – 1 teaspoon

Water - .5 cup

Black pepper, ground - .25 teaspoon

The Instructions:

1. Press the tofu, either in a tofu press or between some paper towels and heavy objects (such as kitchen plates) in order to remove as much liquid as carefully. Once your tofu has been pressed for about ten minutes slice it into large half-inch squares.

2. Pour the olive oil into a large non-stick skillet and allow it to come to hot temperature of medium-high heat until the olive oil begins to shimmer. Place the tofu in the pan, being sure that it is not crowded. You will have to do this in batches. Allow the first side of the tofu to sear until browned, flip, and sear the other side. This should take about ten minutes.

3. Remove the tofu from the pan and continue to cook the remaining tofu.

4. While the tofu cooks combine the remaining ingredients into a large food processor and pulse it until it becomes a thick and chunky marinade. Set aside.

5. Once the tofu has all been seared roughly chop it into quarter-inch pieces. Place it in a large bowl along with the prepared marinade, toss the ingredients together, and allow them to marinate for a minimum of thirty minutes or up to eight hours in the fridge.

6. After the tofu has marinated add it to a large skillet over a temperature of medium-high heat. Add in a one-quarter cup of water and bring the liquid to a simmer. Continue to simmer the tofu until it heated through, about ten minutes.

7. Remove the sofritas from the heat and serve it in taco salad, burritos, tacos, and anything else you might fancy.

Chapter 10:

Frequently Asked Questions

There are many questions people may have when starting the vegan ketogenic diet. In this chapter, we will be answering some of the most common questions, so that you can put your mind at ease and attain success.

Why and How Do I Track My Macro Ratio?
If you hope to maintain ketosis, which is the entire point and a fundamental aspect of the ketogenic diet, you need to track your ketones. Otherwise, you will eat too many carbs to maintain ketosis, eat too little protein to maintain muscle mass, and likely either under eat or overeat fat. You would be surprised how quickly calories from fat and carbs can add up, and you must stay vigilant.

Thankfully, it doesn't have to be difficult to track your macro ratio. There are many diet and health apps that allow you to input amounts of food, and in turn, it calculates the number of calories, carbs, protein, and fat you have eaten. There are many choices of smartphone apps you can use, including Keto Diet App, KetoApp, Carb Manager, and My Fitness Pal.

How much Time does it take to get to Ketosis?
The time required to enter ketosis will vary for each individual. While this can be frustrating, there is a good reason for it. Firstly, a person is unable to enter ketosis until they have burned off all of the glucose and glycogen (a stored version of glucose) within their body. As the body can hold two-thousand calories worth of glucose and glycogen at any given time it will take a while for your body to burn through this glucose. However, if you are someone who is highly active or were already on a moderate carbohydrate diet prior to starting keto then you should enter ketosis within the first day, or at least by the second day. Yet, people who are not

active will take a few days to enter ketosis, as the body will only burn the glucose slowly if the body is not moving around. Lastly, it will take people with insulin resistance the longest amount of time to enter ketosis, requiring about a week. As their bodies don't properly manage glucose it takes more time, but they do enter ketosis eventually. Don't give up hope, just wait a little time and it will naturally happen.

Secondly, once you finally do enter ketosis you will only be in the first stage. During the beginning stages of ketosis, your body will be producing acetone, which is an ineffective ketone. Thankfully, after a week or two of being in ketosis, your body will begin to enter deep ketosis, which is when your body begins to produce acetoacetate and beta-hydroxybutyrate, in the process dumping the excess acetone you no longer need.

Acetoacetate and beta-hydroxybutyrate are much better sources of fuel and better ketones to rely on. It can take a few weeks to fully enter and adjust to the deep ketosis, but it is worth it.

Why Do I Have Headaches and Fatigue?

When adjusting to the ketogenic diet many people will experience headaches, fatigue, insomnia, dry mouth, and more. Overall, it actually feels much like the seasonal flu, yet it is not contagious. What causes this? Put simply, it is known as the "keto flu" and is the body's natural response to adjusting to the ketosis process. The keto flu is due to the body attempting to no longer use glucose for fuel and instead produce its own ketones. These symptoms can be incredibly difficult and frustrating, but thankfully they only tend to last a couple of days or up to a week. The exact length of the keto flu varies from person to person since everyone enters ketosis at a different rate and some people have more difficulty adjusting to changes.

The keto flu is often worsened by dehydration, which is caused when your body dumps excess fluids and water weight. In order to treat your symptoms and manage the keto flu try to stay hydrated with plenty of water paired with the four essential electrolytes. It is commonly recommended to drink half your body's weight of pounds in ounces, meaning that if you weigh two-hundred pounds you will need to drink one-hundred ounces of water daily.

How Many Carbs can I eat and Stay in Ketosis?

The exact number of carbs a person can eat will vary depending on their health, activity level, body type, height, weight, and more. Yet, there is a general rule that you should eat between twenty and twenty-five net carbs, with thirty being the maximum. Any more than this and most people will have too much glucose in their system to maintain ketosis. Although, there are exceptions. People who are highly active and participate in extreme exercising might be able to consume up to fifty net carbs and maintain ketosis, but only if they exercise after eating.

Is the Vegan Ketogenic Diet Maintainable?

The length of time a person chooses to maintain the vegan ketogenic diet is a personal choice. Remember, you don't have to decide beforehand how long you will maintain the lifestyle, simply focus on following the plan one day at a time.

Many people have found vegan and ketogenic diets to be maintainable, with professional scientific studies coming to the same conclusion. There are many people who maintain both the vegan and ketogenic diets for the remainder of their lives.

Is it Possible to Maintain or Gain Weight?

If you are someone who is underweight and looking to gain weight or are already at your ideal weight and hoping to maintain, then you will be happy to know you can do this with the vegan ketogenic diet. Sure, people commonly use it in order to lose weight, but if you follow the plan along with a high-calorie intake you will be able to meet your goals.

In order to maintain or gain weight, you should use a keto macronutrient calculator. This calculator should ask you various things about yourself, including your goals. If you place your goals at either maintaining or gaining weight the calculator will let you know exactly how many calories and macronutrients you need in order to succeed.

Conclusion

You now fully understand the vegan ketogenic diet, allowing you to implement it in your life in a simple and easy to manage manner. This will be especially simple to follow when you implement the meal planning and prepping.

There is no reason to hold back, not when you can receive health benefits, weight loss, increased energy, satisfaction, improve the environment, and much more. It takes time to adjust to the vegan ketogenic diet. While some people can jump in head first overnight, others may take a month to adjust, and that is okay! Feel free to follow the vegan and ketogenic lifestyle at your own pace, you will eventually get to where you want to be.

CPSIA information can be obtained
at www.ICGtesting.com
Printed in the USA
BVHW010443131020
590816BV00026B/1135